Springer Series on
LIFE STYLES AND ISSUES IN AGING

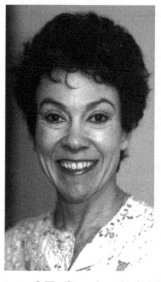

Carole Cox, Ph.D., is Associate Professor at the Graduate School of Social Service, Fordham University. Her previous gerontological work and research have focused in the areas of caregiving, ethnicity, and service utilization, including international comparisons of programs. Dr. Cox is the author of numerous book chapters and articles dealing with various aspects of the issues confronting older persons and their families. Her previous books include *Home Care: An International Perspective* (co-author, Abraham Monk), *The Frail Elderly: Problems, Needs and Community Responses,* and *Ethnicity and Social Work Practice* (co-author, Paul Ephross). She is also the editor of *To Grandmother's House We Go and Stay* (Springer Publishing). Her interest in custodial grandparents and the particular problems they face stems from her personal involvement with these grandparents both in grandparent groups and in the community.

Empowering Grandparents Raising Grandchildren

A Training Manual For Group Leaders

CAROLE B. COX, PhD

 Springer Series on Life Styles and Issues in Aging

Springer Publishing Company, Inc.
536 Broadway
New York, NY 10012-3955

Acquisitions Editor: Bill Tucker
Production Editor: J. Hurkin-Torres
Cover design by James Scotto-Lavino

00 01 02 03 04 / 5 4 3 2 1

Library of Congress Cataloging-in-Publication Data

Empowering grandparents raising grandchildren : a training manual
  for group leaders / Carol B. Cox.
      p. cm. — (Springer series on life styles and issues in aging)
  Includes bibliographical references and index.
  ISBN 0-8261-1316-8 (softcover)
  1. Grandparents as parents.   2. Grandparents—Counseling
  of.   3. Grandparent and child.   4. Grandparenting.   5. Grandchildren—Care.   I. Cox, Carole B.   II. Series.
  HQ759.9.E455   2000
  649'.1—dc21   99-058546
                                                                 CIP

Printed in the United States of America

Contents

Preface

This manual provides a curriculum to be used in groups working towards empowering grandparents who are raising their grandchildren. The training focuses on strengthening the parenting skills of these grandparents so that they are better able to cope with the many challenges they face, both within their homes and within society.

The importance of empowerment training rests in the fact that its effects are not limited to the individual participants. Its effects are also reflected in the communities in which these participants live. Thus, the manual offers training materials for helping grandparents to become active advocates and resource persons for others struggling with the same concerns and needs.

Empowerment training, as presented here, is not intended to replace support groups. In fact, in order to best meet the needs of grandparent caregivers, both types of groups should be offered simultaneously. Having support groups available assures that issues brought up in the training may be explored in greater depth in a more appropriate setting. Indeed, it is difficult to adhere to the training curriculum while exploring the many issues and responses that specific topics may raise.

This training manual is organized into fourteen sessions. These may be reordered, revised, and expanded upon according to the concerns and interests of the individual group. Groups in specific geographic regions or working with distinct ethnic populations may want to add additional material pertinent to their needs.

Brochures and other hand-outs can be valuable adjuncts to the teaching. Obtaining materials from local agencies and programs can help to make the classes more relevant to specific groups. In addition, as participants begin giving presentations or doing outreach in the community, these materials can be distributed.

Finally, this manual should serve as a basis for the further empowering of grandparent caregivers. The development of appropriate and sensitive policies and services congruent with their needs requires a wide range of activities and interventions. This training provides a framework from which grandparents can effectively work towards these needed changes. However, throughout the empowerment process, it is essential to remember that the grandparents themselves are the experts and that they are playing critical roles in the lives of their families, their grandchildren, and society. By helping to further empower them, we all benefit.

Acknowledgments

The initial training was implemented with the members of the Grandparents Empowerment Movement of the Harlem Interfaith Counseling Service, Inc., in New York City. Those participating in the training were: Celestine Grant (Chairperson), Elizabeth Bolling, Gwendolyn Bryant, Johnnie Hooks, Catherine Larry, Maggie Lee, Arlene Miller, Martha Mizell, Normadine Portlett, Gladys Powell, Alice Ryer, Alice Thomas, Alma Warren, and Doris Williams. I am truly indebted to their enthusiasm and interest and remain in awe of their ceaseless spirit, concern, and humor.

The program could not have happened without the vision and leadership of Gwendolyn Florant, Director of the Harlem Interfaith Counseling Service and facilitator of the Grandparents Empowerment Movement. Her belief in the power of the grandparents created an invaluable basis for the project. Special appreciation is given to Sarah Panepinto, graduate assistant, who was able to calmly meet the daily challenges involved in setting up a new program.

I would also like to thank Barbara Draimin, Director of The Family Center, in New York City, who acted as a consultant to the project. Her extensive experience and background in assisting children and families coping with illness, loss, and transitions, made valuable contributions to the curriculum.

The project would not have been possible without the support of the New York Community Trust. This project reflects the interest, concern, and commitment of the Trust to the citizens of New York.

Introduction: Project Description and Guidelines

E mpowerment training seeks to develop self-reliance and foster the ability for self-help. It aims to encourage self-efficacy as it builds upon participants' innate strengths. Consequently, empowerment is congruent with the needs of custodial grandparents. Rather than simply offering assistance or support, it aims to enhance the parenting ability and to assist grandparents to become advocates for themselves and their grandchildren. In addition, the effects of empowerment are not limited to the participants themselves. For, as they become empowered, they impact the very communities in which they live, both as resources and as models for others.

The Empowerment Process

Goals of empowerment practice are helping clients to achieve a sense of personal power, to become more aware of connections between individual and community problems, to develop helping skills, and to be able to work collaboratively towards social change (Gutierrez, 1990). Among the many definitions of empowerment are: the ability to influence people, organizations, and the environment affecting one's life (Cochran, 1987; Hasenfeld, 1987); gaining, developing, seizing, enabling, or giving power (Staples, 1990); and attaining control over one's life, including further participation in the community (Berger & Neuhaus, 1977; Katz, 1984).

According to Gutierrez and Ortega (1991), the personal level of empowerment is concerned with the individual's feelings of personal power and self-efficacy, while the interpersonal level is concerned with an individual's ability to influence others. Practical knowledge, information, real competencies, concrete skills, material resources, genuine opportunities, and tangible results are necessary for empowerment to be developed and sustained (Staples, 1990). Once sustained, the empowered individuals benefit the entire community (Lee, 1994).

Grandparents in the parenting role are often overwhelmed by the problems of their children, grandchildren, and the social milieu in which they live. Economic insecurity, little access to information, lack of training, and physical and emotional stress are factors that contribute to feelings of powerlessness. These feelings are magnified by encounters with complex and difficult systems which they suddenly need for assistance and with which they may be totally unfamiliar.

Empowerment Strategies

Strategies to foster empowerment generally are practiced with groups. Within the group, participants are able to share concerns, learn from each other, and practice specific parenting techniques as well as those related to their roles in the community. As participants become comfortable with these techniques, they are encouraged to use them in other settings. Role-playing and the use of videos as participants try out new behaviors are important strategies for teaching and reinforcing new behaviors.

Throughout the group process the leader acts as a facilitator, recognizing that the participants are the experts and that they will learn best from each other. Helping the participants to begin by solving small problems on their agenda offers a basis for reassuring them of their abilities to solve larger ones and of their own effectiveness. It is important to remember that the role of the group leader is that of a facilitator, rather than an expert. The leader must recognize that the participants learn best from each other and from understanding that their problems are not unique.

The Training Sessions

Curriculum Development

This curriculum developed out of the needs and interests of a group of African-American grandparents in New York City. Prior to the development of the course, informal discussions were conducted with the group and their facilitator to highlight topics that would be most interesting and useful. These discussions shaped the curriculum underscoring immediate concerns and areas where empowerment could be particularly relevant.

Participants received the complete curriculum at the first session. This included all of the class outlines, notes, and materials. In addition, brochures were handed out whenever applicable. Resource material on local legal programs and service agencies that the grandparents may need is particularly useful. In addition, brochures and information on subjects such as HIV/AIDS, sex, and parenting issues are also available from many government and non-profit agencies.

Class Format

Each class involved a variety of teaching techniques with lecture kept to a minimum. With the goal being empowerment, it is essential that the facilitator not be perceived as the expert (Gutierrez, 1990; Lowy & O'Connor, 1986). The grandparents were expected to be active participants and discussion was encouraged. At the same time, achieving a balance between discussion and presentation can be difficult. Participants enjoy relating their own personal experiences with regard to much of the material. Although this helps to reinforce the learning, it also diverges from the curriculum and thus needs to be limited.

The classes focused on developing knowledge, skills, and behaviors, and demanded a great deal of interaction among the participants as they worked to apply the material to their own lives. These interactions also invoked much reflection as the participants were asked to continually question and critique themselves. This type of active learning is critical to the learning process.

Each class involved a variety of teaching techniques with lecture kept to a minimum. Videos were used in several of the classes and were extremely helpful with topics such as communication, loss, and understanding children's ways of expressing grief.

The classes were three hours each and were given at a university, with transportation provided for the participants. The setting was an important part of the empowerment training as it helped to familiarize the participants with environments outside of their community. In addition, attending classes at a university was in itself an "empowering" experience appreciated by the grandparents.

The sessions were held twice a week and participation was mandatory. If participants missed as session, they remained responsible for learning the material. Missing more than two sessions meant that the person was dropped from the training. As a means of reinforcing the learning, and also as a means of increasing grandparents' comfort in making presentations, members in the group were responsible for sharing the material of the missed session with the grandparent. This technique was highly effective as participants were eager to show what they had learned.

At the end of each class, the grandparents completed brief evaluations describing how much they felt they had learned and what was most and least important. Unlike many students, the group tended to write that "everything was important," and that what they really wanted was more time. The entire course was evaluated at the last session.

Role-Playing

Role-playing was used in each class. As most of the participants were unfamiliar with the technique, it was at first greeted with trepidation. But, as the group became familiar with it, they became increasingly enthusiastic and less self-conscious, often enacting the roles with a great deal of humor.

The technique was particularly helpful in assisting the grandparents in dealing with sensitive and difficult situations. Role-plays of talking to grandchildren about sex and HIV or about the loss of their parents help grandparents to feel more at ease with the subjects. Role-playing within the group helps to reduce tension around sensitive issues.

Role-playing is also important in the learning of new skills. As examples, very successful role-plays involved reinforcing a grandchild's self-image and self-esteem, and rehearsing strategies for dealing with rude or unhelpful agency staff. As well as trying out new techniques, the role-plays enabled the participants to gain further insight into the other's role. In addition, the expertise of several of the grandparents in specific situations contributed to learning new behaviors.

Presentations

As the goal of this empowerment training is developing the participants into community advocates and resource persons, each grandparent was required to give a short presentation on a subject covered in the curriculum. This activity, which was feared by many, had very positive results. However, it is important that the setting in which the presentations are given is non-threatening and supportive. Thus, within the group, the participants highlighted what was good in each presentation while also noting where some improvement was needed. Speaking for a few minutes on subjects that they were interested in and had prepared for was another empowering tool.

Assignments

Homework assignments were given as a further means of reinforcing the learning. They also indicated how useful the material was. As part of their assignments, participants were required to use some of the learning each week at home and to report on the outcomes.

The group was very enthusiastic about the use of a "feelings thermometer," which was introduced in the first session as a way of appraising both their own and their grandchildren's temper and emotions. It was also referred to in the sessions as way of indicating whether participants were getting too aggressive or conversely, were losing interest and becoming lethargic.

The grandparents found the thermometer very useful in assessing their interactions with their grandchildren. It helped both parties to recognize any tension that could be affecting their actions. In some instances, the grandchildren themselves began to refer to the thermometer when dealing with their grandparents, particularly when they felt annoyed.

Each grandparent was also asked to keep a journal in which conversations or events related to the classes could be recorded. If they felt comfortable and felt that something had occurred that was pertinent to the learning, they were asked to share what they had written with the group.

Graduation

After the completion of the twelve sessions, a graduation ceremony was held at the University with grandparents inviting their grandchildren, relatives, and friends. The formal event was a further reinforcement of the training, as well as a recognition of the accomplishment of the grandparents. The Dean of the School and others in the community who were involved with both city government and grandparent programs attended, with several making presentations. As the grandmothers received their diplomas, their grandchildren accompanied them onto the stage. The event publicly validated the group's efforts and achievement and served as another source of empowerment.

Support Group

The grandparents continued to attend a support group throughout the training. Having this group was an important adjunct to the classes, as it meant that personal experiences and problems, which were frequently alluded to during classes, could be referred to this group. Given the nature of the training and its relevance to the lives and concerns of the grandparents, it would be difficult to adhere to the class curriculum without this separate support group, where feelings and problems, raised in the training, could be expressed. By assuring that separate counseling and support are available to participants, the training is able to remain focused.

Project Outcomes

With the completion of the training, the grandparents began their on-going task of reaching other grandparents in the community. They were responsible for giving presentations to groups at schools, senior centers, churches, tenant associations, and in other settings in which grandparents and other caregivers were located. Initially, the facilitators played major roles in scheduling these presentations, with the grandparents themselves eventually assuming the responsibility. Follow-up trainings were scheduled periodically to review the presentations and provide further assistance.

The presentations were made in groups of two or three with each grandparent deciding on a specific topic. One of the group facilitators attended the first presentations as a means of offering support and determining the areas where further training was needed. Thus, it was noticed that the grandparents had difficulties in ending presentations, and consequently a follow-up session focused on closings and taking audience questions. Another session addressed the importance of knowing the interests of the audience and their backgrounds to assure that the material was relevant to the specific group.

Guidelines

The following guidelines may assist in the implementation of the training:

1) Be sure that the material is clear and understood by all participants.
2) Make sure the expectations and goals of the training are clear to all participants.
3) Keep the classes focused, do not permit too much digression.
4) Make sure that all participants have the opportunity to talk.
5) Encourage discussion and participation.

6) It is important to keep a balance between lecture and discussion, as participants do want to hear from the "experts."

7) Encourage and use role-play in every session.

8) Develop a resource file of materials for the classes.

9) Have a separate support group available for the participants so that they can further discuss issues and concerns raised in the classes.

10) Use videos as they can be important resources in the training.

11) Keep a sense of humor and to create a relaxed atmosphere.

12) Remember, the grandparents are the experts; the group leader is there to enhance their skills and provide information but must be careful not to dominate the sessions or act as if he/she has all the answers.

Session 1

Understanding Empowerment

OUTLINE

A) Introductions
B) Session objectives
C) Purpose and course structure
D) 1. Explanation of empowerment
    2. Empowerment within the family
    3. Empowerment within the community
E) Prochaska's Stages of Change
F) Activities

Session 1

Understanding Empowerment

W hat does it mean to be empowered and why is it important? Empowerment is important to the well-being of every person. Many are empowered and never even know it, while others feel a lack of power. They feel that they have no control over anyone, over their situations or even over themselves. These classes are meant to enhance your abilities as grandparents and to assure your sense of empowerment. This empowerment takes place in the home, in your families, and in the community.

Objectives

At the end of this session, participants will be able to:

1) Describe why empowerment is important to everyone.
2) Discuss factors which can cause people to feel a lack of power.
3) Identify ways to help grandparents become empowered.

Purpose and Structure of the Course

The purpose of this twelve-session training course is not only to help you to improve your skills as a grandparent, but to also prepare you to work with other grandparents in the community who are also raising their grandchildren. In each three-hour session, we will be presenting you with material which you can use in your own home with your own grandchildren. But, we will also be working towards having this material in a form which you can use in talking to others, either in groups or individually.

Throughout the course, your participation, suggestions, and criticisms will be very important. We need your feedback to make the course really usable and as valuable as possible.

1) Each class will be three hours and will include much discussion and lots of time for you to practice the material on each other.
2) Even though there is a lot of material to cover, the classes should be *fun*. We want this to be enjoyable and that means laughter is important.
3) Everything in the class that concerns your own lives should be kept confidential and shouldn't be discussed with others outside of the classes.
4) This is not the same as a support group and is not the place to discuss your problems in detail since we won't be able to solve them here. That needs to be saved for your counseling group.
5) At the end of each session, we will be asking you to tell us what you liked about the class and what you did not like. This will be very helpful to the development of the program.

Feelings Thermometer

In order to accomplish everything that needs to be done in each class, we are going to use a feelings thermometer. Think of this as measuring feelings in our group. When feelings get really hot and strong the comfort level in the room will be poor. That is when the thermometer will be very high and it will be difficult to work. (These thermometers can be made with construction paper.)

The comfort level is best for learning when the thermometer isn't too high or too low. A really low thermometer means things are really boring!!

Each of us should be aware of the temperature in the group and if things get really hot, someone should call for *"Time Out."* At the same time, if things get really slow and start to drag, someone needs to say *"Get Moving."*

Empowerment

Everyone goes through stages in their lives when they feel more or less powerful, more or less in control of their lives and their circumstances.

- Most young people have a sense of endless power, that they can do anything and that they have all the time in the world to do it in.
- As people grow older, this sense of power often grows less, particularly when circumstances get out of control.
- Becoming a parent again, late in life, taking on the responsibilities of raising grandchildren, can make even the most "powerful" become doubtful about themselves and their abilities.
- A major factor affecting powerlessness is not having the resources necessary for solving problems. These resources are both the knowledge and the skills which enable people to work effectively to influence or change the things which are bothering or oppressing them.

As grandparents, empowerment may involve:

- Being able to feel comfortable in parenting your grandchildren, knowing that you are raising them well and that they are listening to you and becoming stronger, responsible people.
- The way you interact with schools, agencies, services, government officials, and all those who affect the programs and benefits you receive and should receive. Being able to act in a way to assure that you and your grandchildren receive everything to which you are entitled is what is meant by empowerment.
- Empowerment also concerns your relations with others in the same situation as you. By being empowered, you can help other

grandparents to achieve the same goals that you seek, whether they are more benefits, changes in laws, or new community services.

- Working together can be the most *empowering* of all since it can give you the greatest control over your lives. Moreover, helping others to become empowered further empowers you.

One of the most important factors in becoming empowered is learning how to communicate effectively so that your needs are understood and you are able to understand the needs of others. Throughout the course, communication and listening skills will be stressed. You can use these skills with each other, with your grandchildren, and with other grandparents in the community.

Empowerment in Your Family

Empowerment within your family generally means that people listen to you, that you are respected, and that you feel that both your needs and those of your relatives are being met. As grandparents raising grandchildren, you may feel very *"unempowered."* These feelings are likely to happen when you feel that you are being taken advantage of, or that you have little control over your own life or that of your children or grandchildren.

1) Think about situations in which you felt a lack of power within your family.
2) Think about situations in which you felt empowered.
3) What differences were there between the situations in which you felt a lack of power and those in which you felt empowered?

Empowerment in the Community

Empowerment within the community means that you are able to get the services that you feel you need, that you know where to go for assistance if you do not receive them, and that you are able to assist others to get the same services. Being empowered in the community means being aware of your rights and knowing what to do if your rights are violated. It means being able to solve a problem by knowing how to reach the right people and having them listen to you.

1) Think about situations in which you felt a lack of power within the community.
2) Think about situations in which you felt empowered.
3) What differences were there between the situations in which you felt a lack of power and those in which you felt empowered?

The Stages of Change

Change is never easy. Think about how difficult it is to lose weight, stop smoking, or start exercising. The same is true with empowerment. It is best to think of it as a process that occurs in stages. The following model can be helpful as you begin this training (Prochaska, DiClemente, & Norcross, 1992).

Prochaska's Stages of Change

No Problem (Precontemplation): "I don't have any problem with my grandchild"

- I don't have a problem
- Want everyone else to change (teacher, parent, partner)
- Have self-defeating behavior that is demoralizing

Getting Ready (Contemplation): "I should do something about her behavior"

- I want to stop feeling so stuck
- Struggling to understand the problem
- Not yet ready to change
- Substitute thinking about change for actually making a change

Getting Set (Preparation): "I'll start correcting her next week"

- I will stop next week
- Last minute resolution

- Still ambivalent about moving ahead to act
- Begin changing self image (I am in control)

Action: "When she talks back, she will take 'time out.' "

- Overtly modifying behavior
- Action does not equal change
- Begin changing activities and environment

Maintenance: "Every time she talks back, she knows what the result will be."

- Consolidate and maintain gains
- Prevent relapses

Termination: "My grandchild no longer misbehaves."

- There is no problem anymore and there never will be
- There is no temptation or threat

Activities

---

1) Role-play an *empowered* grandparent dealing with a teen-age grandchild, an adult child, and an agency person who doesn't seem to want to listen.
2) Each person makes a presentation to the group about what it means to be empowered and why it is important.

Session 2

Helping Children Build Self-Esteem

OUTLINE

A) Review of last session
B) Session objectives
C) The importance of self-esteem
D) Ways to promote self-esteem
E) What to say/what not to say
F) The importance of "listening" and "hugs"
G) Activities

Session 2

Helping Children Build
Self-Esteem

S elf-esteem is the value that we place on ourselves. Children who are treated with respect, love, and guidance learn that they are valuable people and develop high levels of self-esteem. On the other hand, children who have been neglected, abused, treated poorly, or ignored learn that they have little value and consequently, may have very poor self-esteem.

Objectives

At the end of this session, participants will be able to:

1) Describe three reasons why self-esteem is important.
2) Discuss reasons why their grandchildren may have problems with self-esteem.
3) Describe four ways for increasing their grandchildren's self-esteem.

The Importance of Self-Esteem

Self-esteem is important, as it means feeling worthwhile and valued. Children with good self-esteem feel in control of their lives and have a sense of power. Children who lack self-esteem are much more likely to be influenced by others who they feel are more powerful and important. Competent children see themselves as successful and are able to do better in school, in relationships, and in work.

Children who are being raised by their grandparents are often likely to have lower feelings of self-esteem. Many times they have been abused or neglected and rejected by their parents. By the time they come to their grandparents, they may feel that they have little value or importance. Those who feel that they were abandoned have little trust in adults. If they did not feel protected or secure with their parents, it will be difficult for them to trust in their grandparents.

Often, these children are unable to relax and stay watchful and self-protective. Learning to trust the grandparents can take a long time and requires a lot of patience from the grandparents. Children may feel they have to test you time after time before they really believe you. This can be very tiring. Simply telling children something and expecting them to believe it is not enough, children need explanation and practice.

Building Trust

It is important to be patient and to understand that your grandchildren may need a lot of reminders from you before they can really feel secure and trust you. It is also important to be predictable and consistent.

Follow through on any rules that you have since this makes the child feel secure. If your grandchild knows that you don't like loud music and that every time it gets too loud, you will go in and turn it off, he will begin to feel that he can trust you and the rules. If he begins to trust in this rule and the way you respond, he will eventually begin to trust in you and in the other rules you set. He may not like them, but he will know that the rules are there.

Trust is basic to feeling secure and valuable and is fundamental to positive self-esteem.

Ways to Promote Self-Esteem

1)   Give compliments. Be sure to compliment your grandchild everyday for something they did. Be very specific: "I like the way you dressed yourself today." "I liked the way you helped me today."

2)   At the table, you can have a compliments game—everyone says a compliment to everyone else on what they did that day.

3)   Let children know that you are proud of them. Put their pictures up in the room. Tell them how much you like what they have made.

4)   Make sure your grandchildren know that you love them. Do something with them each day—read to them, draw with them, have a quiet time to talk with them. Hug, hug, hug. Tell them how important they are to you and that you love them.

5)   *Don't criticize or ridicule. If they make a mistake, point out the problem and a way to make things better.* Don't say, "You're so stupid, how could you spill the milk?" This only lowers self-esteem. Instead, say something like, "I think you hit the milk when you reached for the bread; get a cloth and wipe it up."

6)   Really listen to what your grandchildren are saying. Look at them when they are talking. Even if it is nonsense to you, it is important to them. Your listening helps to make them feel worthwhile. Ask them questions and comment on what they are saying, *even* if you're not sure what it is all about.

7)   Respond to broken rules. Tell your grandchild exactly what he or she did: "You hit your sister. I am worried that you might really hurt her. Tell her what you want and why you are angry at her." When you respond like this, you are telling the child exactly what he did wrong, why it is wrong, and what else he could do. This is much better than screaming, or hitting the child yourself. If you react like that, you aren't telling the child what behavior is wrong or why. If he continues to hit his sister, you must be consistent in the way you respond. Make him leave the room, sit alone at the table or lie down.

8) Hitting or using force will only reinforce bad behavior. Spanking a child and then expecting him not to hit others is very confusing. The same thing is true for yelling and screaming at the child. Children will model behavior after you so it is important that you act the way you want your grandchild to behave.

9) Spend time with your grandchildren. Do activities together—coloring, playing cards, listening to music. This helps the child to believe that he or she is special and important to you. It builds a relationship and trust between you and your grandchild.

10) Make sure your grandchildren know that what they do is important to you. Everyday ask them about their activities and what they did. Visit the school, go to sports events, school meetings, parents' days, and church activities with them.

11) *Do* say things that build self-esteem. "Thank you for helping me in the kitchen, I was feeling really tired and it really made me feel better." "I like the way you cleaned the room, you did a really great job!"

12) *Don't* say things that hurt self-esteem. "Why are you so dumb?" "You look really ugly." "Can't you do anything right?"

13) Give children rewards. When something is done well, be sure to *praise.* Giving them more responsibility is also an important way of giving rewards. If your grandchild always comes home on time, you might reward her by letting her stay out a little later. This increases responsibility and helps to let them know that they are appreciated and trusted.

It is important to focus on your grandchildren's strengths rather than their faults. *Remember,* they are already suffering because, for whatever reason, they can't be with their parents. You can build up their self-confidence by reinforcing their strengths, good behavior and actions. Don't emphasize their weak points or problems.

Be sure to accept your grandchildren as they are, even when they make mistakes. They need to feel secure that your love is always there; this will help to believe in themselves. At the same time, every time they do something right or try to do something right, show them that you recognize and appreciate it.

When you disagree with your grandchildren, tell them why. Everyone disagrees and everyone has different opinions. Be sure you show respect to your grandchildren even though you disagree with them.

This helps to prove to them that they are important, which strengthens their self-confidence and self-esteem.

Activities

---

1) Discuss why self-esteem is so important to children and to all of us.
2) Role-play what you might say to a young child who has just spilled milk all over the floor.
3) Role-play what you might say to a teenager who feels really unhappy about her looks.
4) Talk to the group about three important ways to create self-esteem in children.

Sessions 3 and 4

Communicating with Children

OUTLINE

A) Review of last session
B) Session objectives
C) Listening
D) Each child is different
E) Painful news
F) Secrets
G) Deciding how much to tell
H) Activities

Sessions 3 and 4

Communicating with Children

Because there is so much information to discuss with regard to communicating with children, this topic will be covered in two sessions. This will give time for several role-plays, exercises, discussion, and videos. You might want to start Session 4 at the "Secrets" section.

Talking is one of the many ways we communicate with children. We also communicate with our bodies, as well as by example. In fact, children often wonder why adults tell them to do things that they don't do themselves. When children ask questions such as "What is dead?" or "Where do people go when they die?" or "Why doesn't my mother (father) visit me?" they want clear and direct answers. It is often difficult to communicate clearly even when we want to. Increasing your comfort with talking to children and learning new communication techniques is very important.

This session helps the grandparent assess the family's communication style. It also examines the issue of whether or not to disclose information about a grandparent or parent's health status or illness.

Objectives

At the end of this session, participants will be able to:

1) Assess the grandparent's and child's current situation with regard to communicating.

2) Demonstrate techniques to open communication.
3) Understand the burdens of secrecy and the risks and benefits of disclosing secrets.
4) Describe the importance of ongoing dialogue, particularly with children, after initial discussions.
5) Know when to disclose painful news or secrets to grandchildren.

Assessing the Current Situation in the Household—Listening

Many of us tend to talk *at* our children and tell them what to do. Sometimes, we don't really talk *with* them. It is important to find ways that you can exchange thoughts and feelings with your children. Learning to listen to each other is not always easy, but it is very rewarding.

Listening Exercise

1) Listen for three minutes to the person next to you, but interrupt as often as you like.
2) Listen for three minutes without nodding or smiling or wincing. Do not say anything or interrupt in any way.

What does it feel like to be an interrupted talker? What does it feel like to be a neutral listener who doesn't interrupt?

Often, in our conversations we encourage people to talk, or we manage to stop them. This can happen without our even thinking about it.

Following is a list of conversation starters and stoppers. We'll call them door openers and door slammers.

Door Openers—these encourage grandchildren to talk to you; they start communication.

What do you think?

This is how I feel.

That's a good question.

I don't know but let's find out.

Door Slammers—these discourage talking and communication.

You are too young to understand.

None of your business.

I don't care what your friends are doing.

We'll talk later.

Each Child Is Different

Just as adults differ, so do children. Some children talk continually, while others are very quiet. Teenagers can become withdrawn and silent, retreating to their own rooms or to the telephone. It is very normal for teenagers to talk a lot around their friends and to be quiet around you.

Discussing certain issues like why someone died or why they got ill can be difficult because we are not sure about the answer. Often, children will ask questions for which there are no answers, or ones that are hard to explain. You can always answer, "I wonder . . . "—that validates the question and lets the child go on. You can always say, *"I don't know, what do you think?"*—that is helpful when you are not sure what the child is really asking and also encourages the child to talk about it.

Children will often NOT ask you questions that they think will make you feel bad or uncomfortable. That means that YOU need to create an open and free space for them to have the courage to ask questions. They have to believe that you will respond with a *door opener* rather than a *door slammer*.

For example, a young child may say, "What does sex mean?" You can do one of two things. You can try to answer what you believe and what you think the child can understand, or you can start by assessing where the child is at, by asking questions such as "What do you think?" or "That's a good question; what led you to ask me that question?"

When we jump too quickly to answer children's questions, we sometimes miss what they were really trying to learn or tell us. Give some examples of this from your own grandchildren.

Painful News

Painful news is anything that we believe is going to upset the grandchild. It may be about their parent, yourself, their future, or anything that affects them and their well-being.

When you have to share painful news, it is good to begin by thinking about your grandchild's strengths and previous reactions.

It is very common for children to act out in some way, by misbehaving or becoming withdrawn, particularly when they hear news about their parent. Think about how your grandchild has responded to painful news.

It is quite common for children to respond to bad news with temporary behavioral problems. When you are speaking with your grandchildren you can say to them that they might find it a little harder to concentrate in school or that they might feel angry without knowing why. Tell them that this is normal and that you want to know about it when it happens.

One of the most common responses from children is a delayed reaction to their grandparent's news. Upon hearing about illness, children will often not seem upset or even ask any questions. Grandparents can interpret this to mean that the children don't care. Clearly this is not the case—*Children need time,* as do adults, to adjust to this type of news. A child may take days before they show their reaction, but they will have one eventually. *You need to pay close attention to any signs of depression or changes in behavior.*

A child's initial reaction to "news" may also change over time:

Younger children sometimes return to behaviors they had outgrown, such as bed-wetting or thumb-sucking.

Older children may hide their feelings, withdraw, or act out as a way of expressing sorrow or anger.

Adolescents may engage in risky behavior, such as drug use or sexual experimentation.

Some children will become extremely protective of their grandparents.

When a person considers talking to children about an illness, there are some special considerations that need to be kept in mind.

Age, for example, dictates the type of language a grandparent uses in order to explain things about the diagnosis. In order to help a child feel less anxious, grandparents need to carefully choose words, especially when they are talking to their younger children.

The grandparent can "set the stage" for talking with their grandchildren:

Where do your children feel most comfortable?

Do you have a special place where you like to have serious conversations?

When is the best time to sit and talk to your grandchildren?

Do you have a weekly "talk time" or chat corner?

Secrets

Assessing Readiness to Disclose Secrets

Families and grandparents often have "secrets." These are matters that they do not like to share either with their relatives or outside of the family. However, keeping secrets can be difficult and may not be in the best interest of the grandchild. At the same time, deciding to tell someone else about a private matter is a personal choice. It is up to you to decide when and how to talk to your friends and family about an issue. No one should be telling you how to handle this situation.

Do you have any issues you find difficult to discuss with your grandchildren? Examples might be why they are not living with their parent or what happened to their parent.

Has your child talked to you directly about drug use or an HIV diagnosis? What was your reaction?

Did you find out another way? How did you feel?

What have you told your grandchildren directly about their parent's situation? What was their reaction?

Evaluating the Pros and Cons of the Decision to Disclose

Some people find that disclosing personal information to others helps them accept themselves and move forward with their lives. They receive additional help and support from friends and family. Others are more reluctant to reveal information for a variety of reasons, including rejection from friends, family or their community.

Deciding to tell people your "secrets" requires you to consider and balance many factors.

The Burdens of Secrecy

Everyone has a right to keep his or her business private, but some people feel relieved after they are open with friends and family. Can you imagine anyone who has been worried about you who might feel relieved to know the truth? Can the truth help people to feel closer to you and more important in your life?

While the reluctance to disclose "secrets" may be based partly on the desire to protect others from pain or from rejection, keeping a secret can create stress in a family. For example, young children can often sense when something is wrong, especially if their parent or grandparent is ill. When they have no information about the problem, they often make up their own stories to explain what they observe, and because there is no one to talk with, children keep these ideas to themselves. Holding onto this type of fear is very stressful for young people. CHILDREN OFTEN FEEL THAT A "SECRET" IS THEIR "FAULT."

Maintaining Secrets with Children

It can be very difficult for children to keep secrets. Children, in particular, may inadvertently tell others.

It can be upsetting, especially for children, to learn from someone else that their parent or grandparent is/was sick. In particular, teenagers may feel as if their grandparent has not respected them enough to speak with them directly.

Is it important to think about what your children or friends/ family know?

Have you ever told your children something personal about yourself and asked them not to discuss it? Were they able to respect your privacy?

How important is it that you limit the number of people who know about your secret?

Do you have a child who just cannot keep a secret?

Do you feel awkward asking a child to keep a secret?

Deciding How Much to Tell

There are many levels of telling, especially if it is about an illness. One can begin with: a person has an illness; continue with: this illness is serious; to: the illness is terminal; and finally: the specific nature of the illness. This concrete picture can help people see that they do not have to tell everyone everything, that in fact, they have a variety of options and can tell different people different amounts of information.

Things to consider when talking to children of different ages:

Age two and under: They don't really understand illness. They are more concerned about what is happening to them. Separation from parents is a major worry.

Age two to seven: They are better able to understand things like illness. They believe the world revolves around them. They often think that their behavior caused the problem. If they are just "good," things will get better. Give simple explanations. Expect the same questions and concerns to come up over and over. They need time and repeated assurance.

Age eight to twelve: They are starting to understand relationships among several events. The understanding of death varies among these children. Many in this age group think or worry about dying, but often don't tell anyone.

Age twelve and over: They can usually understand complex relationships between events. They can think about things they have not yet experienced. They like to know details about things like illness.

Ongoing Talks

Children need to know they can talk to you. You should have a set time and safe space when others will not walk in. It is helpful to have a routine talk time. This might be at Friday night dinner, before prayers, after school, or whatever time is best for you and your grandchild.

Activities

---

1) Demonstrate "door openers" and "door slammers."
2) Describe how children may respond to "painful news."
3) Role-play discussing a "secret" with your grandchild.
4) Discuss the subjects that you hesitate to talk about with your grandchild.

Session 5

Dealing with Behavior Problems

OUTLINE

A) Review of last session
B) Session objectives
C) Questions to ask
D) Reasons for misbehavior
E) Punishment and discipline
F) Temper tantrums
G) When to get help
H) Adolescents
I) Activities

Session 5

Dealing with Behavior Problems

Children often have difficulty managing their behavior. All children misbehave from time to time, but it is extra hard to deal with when you are NOT the parent. It is also extra hard when you know that the child wishes the parent were there to take care of them. Parenting as a grandparent raises special challenges.

Objectives

At the end of this session, participants will be able to:

1) Identify and assess the reasons for acting-out behavior.
2) Figure out the right amount of structure and flexibility for their child.
3) Know where to get additional help.

It is important to be as informed as possible about three areas of your grandchild's life. These three areas to look at in assessing your grandchild are school, health and general well-being. It is often good to check out your assessment with teachers and other family members.

Questions to Ask

Following are some of the questions that you should know the answers to.

Questions About Programs or School

What have you heard from the people who are with your child during the day in either day care or school?

What kind of feedback have you gotten from the program?

What kind of feedback do you get from your grandchildren? Are they enjoying themselves—do they leave easily in the morning and come home happy?

Who is your grandchild's best friend? How do they get along with other children their own age?

What would you say is your grandchild's best subject in school? What subject does he/she have the most trouble with?

Questions About Health

What do you know about grandchild's health?

How is your grandchild's appetite?

How are his/her sleeping habits? Does he/she go to bed easily? Can he/she sleep through the night? Does he/she have nightmares? Bedwetting or soiling?

Does she/he get frequent headaches or stomachaches?

When was the last time your grandchild saw a doctor?

General Questions

These questions can help you to further understand your grandchild.

Does your grandchild have any particular fears?

How does your grandchild get angry? Does he/she have any tantrums? How do you handle this? What makes your grandchild angry?

How does your grandchild show happiness? What does your grandchild do when he/she is in a good mood?

Has your grandchild ever gone to therapy? Why did he/she go? What was the result?

Misbehavior

When your grandchild misbehaves, there are two tasks to handle: respond to the child so that he/she stops misbehaving, and teach your child to know and strive for good behavior. These are both easier to say than do.

Children misbehave for three main reasons:

a) They don't know the rules
b) They know the rules but break them anyway. They maybe frustrated, angry, in need of attention or unable to control their desires.
c) They don't feel well because they are sick, hungry, tired, or upset and don't know how to express it.

Your grandchild's world may seem simple to you, but for the child it is often filled with curiosity that leads to trouble, insecurity which leads to anger, frustration because there are so many things to learn, and temptation to reach out and try it all.

To Help Prevent Misbehavior:

a) Set clear rules and routines for bedtimes, meals and getting off to school.
b) Be consistent with your rules and stick to them.
c) Be firm and fair when a child breaks the rules.
d) Be encouraging when your child is behaving well.

e) Give lots of attention for good behavior. Don't take it for granted.

Since all children have slip-ups, be prepared with a few things you can do:

a) Time-outs—Send your child to a safe, quiet place away from people and toys for a few minutes (one rule of thumb suggests 1–2 minutes for each year of your child's age). Time-outs should be used for serious types of misbehavior.
b) Tune Out—Ignore misbehavior that is aimed at getting your attention. Let your child know that you are ready to respond when he or she stops the behavior.
c) Remove Privileges—Take away something the child values such as playtime or a game.

Spanking

There are a lot of different opinions on the pros and cons of spanking. Most professionals believe that it is not a good idea because it does NOT teach a child how to control his or her behavior. Instead, it sends a message that hitting is OK for solving problems.

Differences Between Punishment and Discipline

Discipline teaches a child structure and how to control behavior. *Punishment* is the consequence done to the child for wrong behavior.

To Develop and/or Change Behavior

Start with positive behaviors—reinforce all positive actions that the child does.

Teach children that negative behaviors get negative consequences.

Be specific with your grandchildren.

Include the child in your plan, especially in choosing rewards.

Do your planning when you are both calm.

Make charts and contracts about the behavior.

Respond immediately to the child's actions, both good ones and bad.

Young Children

What About a Temper Tantrum?

Try to prevent tantrums by seeing them coming. They usually occur when a child is tired and is getting more and more frustrated. Ensure the child's safety by removing all objects or moving your child to a non-public place. Let your child know you are ready to respond when he/she gets control and stops the tantrum.

What About Aggressive Behavior Such as Biting or Hitting?

Stop the behavior by stepping in, if necessary, to prevent anyone from getting hurt. Discuss other ways to respond.

Take some slow deep breaths to calm the mind and body.

Have your grandchild start a sentence with "I get angry when you . . ." or "I feel bad when you . . ."

Use a time-out if necessary.

Bad Language—It Is a Common Way to Get Attention

a) Make sure children know which words are OK and which are not.

b) You could respond by ignoring the bad language or by reminding your child of the rules and carrying through with a consequence.

c) Remember that bad language is usually frustration or a call for attention.

Stealing and Lying

Explain that stealing or lying is the wrong way to meet needs and explain the right way. Explain that *their behavior* is bad. That is *not* the same as calling *them* bad. Arrange for return, repayment, or replacement of stolen items. Children need to understand that they must pay for this behavior. Help your child face the facts by your stating the facts. (Don't try to get them to admit wrong-doing or they may lie and get themselves in deeper.)

Talking Back and Saying NO

When a child does this, he or she has a need for control. Try to give them a choice. Say, "Would you like to have a bath first or clean up your room first?" If they keep saying no and talking back, you can ignore the behavior, remind them that you won't bend the rules, or follow through with a loss of privilege.

A Few More Hints

Don't sweat the small stuff. Pick your battles. Buttoning up a sweater or fixing a collar or picking up an item is usually small stuff. If it becomes big, it is because your child is tired, upset, sick, or just trying to get your attention.

Don't expect perfection since we all make mistakes.

Try to cool down before *you* respond in anger. Never belittle your grandchild or call him names. Focus on specific behaviors that need to be changed.

Use the "feelings thermometer" as a means of showing both of you how upset you are.

Seeking Outside Help

When you have tried everything and asked the school and others for feedback, and discipline is not working, *it's time to ask for help.* There are child therapists and counselors who can often help you and a child with problems. They may want to talk to the child alone or with the two of you together. Seeking outside help is not a reflection on you. You and your grandchild have been through a lot. Getting help early can be good for you both.

Adolescents

For a number of reasons the period of adolescence is often the most challenging stage of development for both grandparents and the young person. There are several problems facing grandparents living with adolescents:

1) These young people are frequently more interested in the outside world than life at home.
2) Due to their size, it can be difficult to discipline or restrain them.
3) Adolescents are usually on an emotional roller coaster, changing from happy to angry in seconds.

The general challenge for both grandparents and adolescents is to maintain a reasonably stable home life while allowing the teenager to have some freedom with their peers.

The Complicated Nature of Anger

- Everyone experiences anger. It has many causes: stress, rejection, worry, frustration, loss, fear, etc.
- Anger affects the body: adrenaline, heart pumping, muscles tense, shakiness.

- Handling anger poorly hurts the angry person: damages relationships, health problems, legal trouble, incarceration.
- Handling anger well can help you. Use it as a wake-up call to work through problems and motivate you to change.
- Ignoring anger leads to physical problems: heart problems, high blood pressure, headaches, stomach problems.
- It is important to recognize anger, identify the causes, take a time out and decide what to do.

Activities

---

1) Role-play a response to "bad language" from your grandchild.
2) Describe situations in which you might use "time-out" or "tuning out."
3) Explain the actions you should take when you feel yourself getting angry.

Session 6

Talking with Your Grandchild about Sex and HIV

OUTLINE

A) Review of last session
B) Session objectives
C) The importance of values
D) Talking about sex
E) Talking about HIV/AIDS
F) Activities

Session 6

Talking with Your Grandchild about Sex and HIV

T alking to grandchildren about sex and HIV can be among the most difficult tasks you have. Most grandparents, as well as parents, feel unsure of how to talk about these subjects, as well as when to begin. It is most important to understand the influence that you have on your grandchildren and that this influence is shown most clearly through the guidance you offer. Talking with your grandchildren, showing them the right ways of behaving, and supervising them are particularly necessary.

Objectives

At the end of this session, participants will be able to:

1) Discuss how they can influence the behavior of their grandchildren.
2) Describe ways of talking to their grandchildren about sex and HIV.
3) Demonstrate what to say to a young child and a teenager about HIV and sex.

Your own actions are very important in affecting the behavior of your grandchildren with regard to sex. Children are confronted with pressure from the media and their peers to become sexually active. It is important that you feel able to talk with your grandchildren and that you have started a regular discussion time, which could be once a day or once a week. But having started these regular discussions, it becomes much easier to discuss the more difficult topics of sex and HIV.

You must also be consistent with your grandchildren, when they break a certain rule, even when they are very little, they must know what to expect. This lets children know exactly what the lines of behavior are, what is expected of them, and what will happen when they break the rules. "Time-out," or having the child sit in one place and not play is easy to understand for young children (one minute for each year of age is often suggested). Older children, pre-teens and teens, can be sent to their rooms. *Be sure not to threaten,* just do it. This way the child is really clear about what to expect, and this lays the basic foundation for dealing with the more explosive topics of sexuality and drugs.

Values

Teach your children values and show that you also live by these values. These values are the tools which enable your grandchildren to deal with all the temptations they are likely to meet.

- *Honesty*—Tell the truth; they know when you are lying. If they find out you are lying, why shouldn't they lie?
- *Courage*—Be able to say NO when everyone else is doing it; be able to not follow the crowd.
- *Self-reliance*—Your grandchildren should learn to be responsible for their own actions; learn not to blame others. This means that you also let your grandchildren make decisions for themselves. Learning from their own mistakes is important for developing a sense of responsibility later on.
- *Self-discipline*—Act the way you want your grandchildren to act: not smoking, not drinking alcohol, not cursing, not yelling, not

hitting. Show children proper examples of how you want them to behave.

- *Fidelity*—If you say it, mean it! Be faithful to your commitments. Keep your promises.
- *Justice and mercy*—Be fair; live by the golden rule. If you wouldn't like it to happen to you, don't do it to someone else. Children will see this and learn to live by it themselves.
- *Love*—Teach your grandchildren that you love them, and to love themselves and others. This way they will care what happens to themselves and others.

Remember . . .

Teenagers tend to look most at their friends for models. But, it is important that you continue to be involved and give guidance, encouragement, and discipline. Give lots of praise and let your grandchild earn more independence.

Speak Your Mind

If you don't want your grandchildren to have sexual intercourse, say it. Tell them to wait, that there is time, and that having sex too early can lead to many problems. Set goals for them that they can believe in and let them know you believe in them too.

Listen

Let your grandchildren say what they feel and question your beliefs. This lets them know they can talk to you and express themselves, and can do this without being afraid that you won't love them or that they are doing something wrong. Really try to understand what they are saying and why.

Talking about Sex

Sex is happening earlier and earlier. This means that talking about sex has to begin early; this could be as early as six years old.

a) Think about what you wanted to know when you were a kid. Write it down.
b) Practice what you want to say.
c) Then find the time and place to say it to your grandchild, on the front steps, in the kitchen, wherever you are most comfortable.

At three to five years old, children can understand that men and women have different sex organs. Talk about the way you would talk about teeth or ears; use the right names, vagina and penis. This helps your grandchild to be very clear about your meaning and what you are talking about. It makes the talk honest and this helps your grandchild to open up and have a real conversation. If they ask where babies come from, tell them they grow in a special place inside the mother.

Children in school have usually heard about things like child abuse, rape, and AIDS. So now it is important that you talk about these subjects with them and give them correct information.

Pre-teens are very concerned about fitting in and not being different. They want to be sure that they are normal and accepted. At the same time, this is when it is important to make sure that they "think for themselves" and don't just follow their friends. Most know about or are ready to learn about sexual relationships and now is the time for you to talk with them about diseases like HIV/AIDS, birth control, and the consequences of teen pregnancy. Give them as much information as you think they can understand. What you don't tell them, they are likely to learn on the street, and it is much better if it comes directly from you.

Teens must be able to say "no" and know what is meant by "safe sex." Safe sex lowers the risk of spreading diseases but the safest sex of all is not having it. Teens need to know that *they do not have* to have sex. It is important that they understand that they can refuse sex and that it is their right to do so. It is now that values, self-esteem, and responsibility become most important in their making this decisions.

Birth Control

Teenagers also have to know about birth control. If they choose to have sexual intercourse, then both boys and girls have to know how to prevent pregnancy. Boys have to know what their responsibility is if a girl gets pregnant and girls have to understand the responsibility of being a teenage mother.

Both boys and girls need to understand how contraceptives are used for preventing pregnancy and preventing the spread of diseases such as AIDS. Birth control keeps the egg from being fertilized by the sperm. Latex condoms worn on the penis protect against pregnancy and sexually transmitted diseases including AIDS. Without using protection, a girl has a very high risk of becoming pregnant. Without using a condom, the risk of getting a disease is very high. Condoms are safe and inexpensive and can protect both partners from sexually transmitted diseases. Withdrawal is not reliable because sperm can enter the vagina even before ejaculation. In order to protect against sexual diseases, even when the girl uses another method of birth control, she should insist on the boy wearing a condom.

Talking about HIV/AIDS

Much of the spread of AIDS is now coming from drug use, sharing needles, as well as through sexual intercourse. Teenagers who use drugs are at a higher risk of getting AIDS, as they are also less likely to use birth control.

Very young children don't need to discuss AIDS unless they have been directly affected by it, such as having parents or relatives with the disease. If this has happened, you should tell them that it is a serious disease but that they are not going to get it. Give them as much information as you think they can understand.

Children in school, after age five, can be told that AIDS is caused by a virus but that it is hard to get and that they can't get it from sneezing, holding hands, or drinking water. Listen to the questions being asked so that you can answer them and try to keep your answers simple. You may tell your grandchild that AIDS is passed during sex or through needles used by people taking drugs.

Children in middle school should be given more information about the disease and how it is passed as well as prevented. This is the time to let children know that it comes from sexual intercourse, through IV drug use, and is passed through blood and semen. They need to know that condoms can help in preventing AIDS.

Activities

---

1) Role-play discussing sex and HIV with a young child, pre-teen, and adolescent.
2) Discuss the importance of teaching your child values.
3) Role-play discussing the use of contraceptives with your grand-child.

Session 7

Talking with Your Grandchild about Drugs

OUTLINE

A) Review of last session
B) Session objectives
C) The importance of your own behavior
D) Learning how to talk about alcohol and drugs
E) Signs that your grandchild may be using drugs
F) What to do if he or she is using drugs
G) Activities

Session 7

Talking with Your Grandchild about Drugs

L istening to, looking at, and responding to your grandchildren are important in discussing sex and HIV, and are also important in discussing drugs. Helping your grandchild to know how to make responsible decisions can help them to stay away from drugs, even when "everyone else is doing them." But, in preparation for these talks, you must become comfortable about the topics and knowledgeable about certain facts related to drug use among children. It is important to remember that all children can be tempted to use alcohol or drugs.

Objectives

At the end of the session you will be able to:

1) Describe some ways of improving your ability to talk with your grandchild about drugs.
2) Know how to set and enforce rules about the use of alcohol and drugs.

3) Describe signs that a child may be using drugs.
4) Discuss what to do if a child is using drugs.

Talking with Your Grandchild about Drugs

Many believe that their grandchildren will never become involved with drugs and so they just don't discuss drug use with them. Others are afraid that by talking about drugs, they may be encouraging their grandchildren to use them, while many just don't know what to say or how to say it. Following are some ways to help you talk about the subject:

a) Begin to talk to your children at a young age. Even young children can begin to learn about drugs and the problems they can cause.

b) Always listen carefully to your grandchildren and be aware of what they may *not* be saying.

c) Be ready to talk about sensitive topics. Remember, they may be sensitive to you but not to your grandchild who really wants some answers.

d) If you don't have the answer, don't be afraid to admit it, and let your grandchild know that you will find the answer or that you can find it together.

e) Be very clear in your messages about drugs and alcohol so that your grandchild knows exactly what you think about their use.

f) It is important that you model the behavior that you expect. If your grandchild sees you drinking alcohol or taking drugs, he or she will have a difficult time understanding that it is wrong.

Setting the Stage

a) Help children to know it is OK to be independent and not

do what everyone else is doing. This is important to learn at an early age as it can help them to say they don't want to use drugs.

b) Let your child make as many decisions for him or herself as possible and support those decisions. Young children can decide what to wear or who to play with. As children learn to think for themselves and take responsibility for their decisions, they are better able to make the right decision about drug use.

c) Role-play with your grandchild how to say NO to friends. This can help children to not go along with their friends if they are drinking or using drugs.

Setting and Enforcing Rules

It is important to set strong rules with regard to alcohol and drug use. Children may be easily tempted by others so it is very important that your rules are clear and that they are enforced.

a) Be sure that your grandchild understands the rules and the reasons for them.

b) Be sure that your grandchild knows what the consequences will be if the rules are broken.

c) Be consistent about your rules and what is expected of your grandchild.

d) It is important to start with simple rules when children are very young, like holding hands on the sidewalk or when crossing the street. Knowing that there are consequences for breaking rules will make it easier for them to believe you about rules and drugs when they're older.

Stages for Communicating

Young children, between the ages of about five and eight, can be taught what an illegal drug is and the harm it can do. You can tell them how medicines given by the doctor can help heal people, but how they can also be misused and hurt people. You need to give them the rules that you have about drugs and alcohol. But remember, since they also watch your behavior, what you *do* will be very important. This is a time to practice with your grandchild how to say NO if offered something from a stranger or even by a friend.

Children from ten to twelve years old need specific facts and information. Tell them that marijuana, tobacco, alcohol, inhalants, etc., can have long-term, bad effects on their bodies, particularly when they are growing. Tell them that it really *isn't cool* to take these things. Try to get your grandchildren involved in other activities, like sports, church programs, or youth programs in the community which keep them active and involved.

Early teens are tempted to use drugs because their friends do. Reinforce your own values and rules that such use is unacceptable. Explain that "everyone is not doing it" and that the effects can be very harmful. Know where your grandchildren are and who they are with. Get to know their friends' parents as well as their friends. Keep practicing how to say NO.

High school students need you to continue to talk with them about alcohol and drug use. Try to make sure their time is structured; the hours of 3–6 pm are times when they are most likely to experiment with drugs. The busier the teen is, the less likely to start experimenting. Encourage the teen to get involved in the community, through sports or as a volunteer.

What to Look For

Children may begin to experiment with drugs for many reasons, including how they feel about themselves, how they are getting along with friends, and how they are getting along at home. Signs that they may be using drugs include:

Low grades or poor school performance

Aggressive, rebellious behavior

Being easily influenced by friends

Behavior problems

Withdrawn, depressed behavior

Poor relationships with the family

Lack of interest in usual activities

Changes in eating or sleeping patterns

It is important not to confuse normal teenage dress and acting out behaviors with drug use. Teenagers typically like "strange" hair styles, loud music, and different types of dress as ways of establishing their own identity. Acting this way does not mean that they are using drugs or alcohol.

Why Children Abuse Drugs

To see what it is like—they think that experimenting is harmless.

To be part of the crowd—everyone does it.

They feel lonely or bored.

They want to escape from problems or avoid unpleasant feelings.

They have low self-esteem or feel they have less value than others.

Effects of Drug Use

Drug use can result in permanent physical damage and possibly death. "Abuse" means that more and more drugs are needed to produce effects and this leads to dependence. Without the drug, the user can't function. Concentration, memory, attitudes, and skills can be affected.

Drug use can result in legal trouble—conviction can affect an entire life. Possession of illegal drugs can result in fines or prison.

Drug use results in financial problems—drugs are expensive, and many steal or get involved in other crimes to support their drug use.

Drug use can damage relationships—drugs to the addicted person become more important than relationships with family or friends.

Basic Types of Drugs

1) *Stimulants* include amphetamines and cocaine, which speed up the nervous system.
2) *Depressants* include barbiturates, tranquilizers, and alcohol, which slow down the nervous system.
3) *Hallucinogens* include LSD and PCP, which can cause changes in perception and consciousness.
4) *Narcotics* include heroin, which lower the perception of pain.
5) *Cannabis* includes marijuana and hashish, which affect thinking and behavior.

What to Do

- If you have any doubts or concerns about your grandchild's possible use of drugs, have him or her examined by a physician. It is possible that the changes you see are the result of a physical or emotional illness.
- Signs of drug use include pipes, rolling papers, small medicine bottles, eye drops, or butane lighters.
- Don't confront the child if he or she is under the influence of drugs or alcohol—discuss your suspicions or concerns when the child is sober.
- Use whatever discipline you have decided upon when rules are broken.
- Take your grandchild for help—there are many clinics, drug treatment programs, and physicians who evaluate and work with children with drug problems.
- Don't take all the blame on yourself if your grandchild abuses drugs. Deal with the feelings and issues and keep your sanity. Face the problem and do something about it.

Activities

1) Role-play talking to a young child, a pre-teen, and a teenager about drugs.
2) Discuss the importance of rules and how to establish them.
3) Describe what to look for if you think your grandchild is using drugs or alcohol.

Session 8

Dealing with Loss

OUTLINE

A) Review of last session
B) Session objectives
C) Each person is different
D) Your own grief
E) Healthy and unhealthy ways of coping
F) Six steps of mourning
G) Complicated grief
H) Getting help
I) Activities

Session 8

Dealing with Loss

G rief and loss usually make us sad. But grief is also an expression of our love. If we lose something and it doesn't matter to us, we were usually not that attached. Mourning the loss of a person is also celebrating the life and time that you had together. Looking forward shows us that the relationship to them will never be the same. It also means that we need to carry inside us feelings and thoughts that we liked to share. Looking backward is an opportunity to honor what we had and did together. It is a way to give respect and homage to our relationship. It is also a time to examine any regrets that we may have.

Objectives

At the end of the session you will be able to:

1) Describe how people cope with and learn from change and loss.
2) Discuss the different ways in which people may react to loss.
3) Discuss the concept of complicated grief.
4) Appreciate the role of symbols and rituals.

Each Person Is Different

Grief and mourning are as individual as fingerprints. Loss and grief are in proportion to our own scale . . . not anyone else's. Sometimes a person loses a bracelet and becomes unglued. We can't begin to understand why. The bracelet may have a special significance that we don't know about. Or perhaps this person may react very strongly to any loss. Sometimes we are even surprised by our own reactions. Grief can feel as though a big wave rolled over our heads and drenched us with tears or sadness.

Some losses are less obvious than others. When a parent is taking drugs and has strong moods and does not pay attention to the children, the children feel the loss of attention. They may all be in the same room, but the children feel the loss of someone who can love them. When parents make promises and don't keep them, the child and the grandparent often feel a loss of "trust."

Think about some of the losses you have experienced or are experiencing. How have you reacted? Sometimes we expect others to have the same grief reaction as we do. But notice how many different ways people react to a funeral. Do you wonder about all the silly things people say when someone has died? They are usually trying to help but they don't know how and they are doing it in their own way. It is hard not to be affected by each other's reactions. We try to make sense out of someone else's reaction even when it is not possible to do so. A person's reaction can even insult us or make us angry.

Grieving

When we know about our own ways of grieving, we are in a better position to help our grandchildren with their grief. Often, grandparents are hesitant to share their feelings because they believe that children need to be protected from sadness and anger. Some grandparents are concerned that if you are sad in front of the children it will make them sad. This may be true, but the children may feel sad already. You can help them by giving them a chance to share their feelings with you.

If your grandchildren become afraid when they see you cry, you can explain that crying has never hurt anyone and that *nothing bad is going to happen*. You can also explain to them that sometimes it is important to show your feelings and that it helps you to feel better. If you are not ready to talk about your own loss in front of your grandchildren, you may feel more comfortable doing so later on, when the feelings aren't so powerful. If your grandchildren are ready to talk and you are not, perhaps you can invite them to talk with a minister or counselor.

Healthy Ways to Cope

Each of us wants to:

1. Know that the loss happened and exactly what happened.
2. Feel the loss.
3. Adapt to the new way of life and rules.
4. Reinvest our energy and move on while remembering.

Things That Can Help You Cope

- Religion
- Exercise
- Work
- Talking

Are there other methods that you use or would recommend? What are the *not* so healthy ways that you cope with loss?

Six "R" Steps in Mourning

1. Recognize the loss.
2. React to the separation.

3. Recollect and re-experience the deceased and the relationship.
4. Relinquish the old attachments to the deceased.
5. Readjust to the "new world" without forgetting the old.
6. Reinvest the emotional energy you had for the loved one in something or someone who can give something back.

Symbols

Symbols and rituals can help people to cope. But, a symbol that helps one person cope can make it more difficult for someone else. Anniversaries, wakes, memorial services, funerals, and burials are all symbols. They celebrate the person who has died and bring others together. This support can be extremely important in helping people to cope with their grief.

Complicated Grief

In life we all have problems that are simpler, and others that are "wicked." A wicked problem usually has lots of strings attached and depends on many people and things to get it solved. Complicated grief is like a wicked problem. It has lots of strings and there are no easy answers. It took a long time to get complicated and it often takes a long time to get resolved.

Complicated mourning is when one cannot progress through the "R" steps. Often the mourning is intense and unrelenting and goes beyond two years. In complicated mourning, one denies and avoids the loss and pain, and tries to hold onto the lost loved one.

There are four high risk factors for complicated mourning:

- Sudden death
- Loss of a child
- Death after an overly lengthy illness (exhaustion and depletion)
- Death the mourner thinks could have been prevented

Signs That Help Is Needed

You or someone you know is stuck in a mourning stage.

There is extreme rage.

There is extreme guilt.

There is much conflict within the mourning due to a love/hate relationship with the deceased.

There is no stop to the mourning; someone thinks the loss was two years ago and it was twenty; someone visits a cemetery every day.

Serious "accidents" and talk of suicide.

There is a lack of reality.

Severe depression and lack of functioning.

Declining physical, emotional and spiritual well-being.

Extreme isolation and alienation from others.

Activities

1) Describe the actions you take to help you cope with loss.
2) Describe some of the behaviors of your friends or relatives in coping with loss.
3) Role-play explaining to a grandchild why you are crying or feeling sad.

Session 9

Dealing with a Child's Grief and Loss

OUTLINE

A) Review of last session
B) Session objectives
C) How children grieve
D) Helping children talk about death
E) Making a "memory box"
F) Activities

Session 9

Dealing with a Child's Grief and Loss

C hildren experience loss and grief, as adults do, in many different ways. Much of how they experience it will relate to their age. It is important to understand their common reactions so that you can be aware of the more complicated responses suggesting that help may be necessary.

Objectives

By the end of this session, participants will be able to:

1) Learn specific information about how children grieve.
2) Become more comfortable with helping children talk or draw about loss.
3) Learn about a "memory box" and other ways to use photos and mementos.

How Children Grieve

We want to help children deal with loss but we often don't know what to say or when to say it. When a child learns of a parent's death and goes outside to play basketball, that is normal. When a child shows no reaction at all, that is normal. When a child gets angry at everyone and everything and says nothing is wrong, that is normal. Each of us has our own way of dealing with loss.

Grieving can be very confusing. One of the trickiest aspects of grieving is that the feelings do not happen all at once in a single period of time. This means that grief can pop up at the sight of a picture, when you hear a song, or even at the change of a season. This is a strange experience for children. They can be sad one minute, and playing the next. Sometimes it can seem like they have forgotten that they have recently suffered a great loss.

Whereas each child has his/her own way of dealing with loss, there are some things common to different age groups and some warning signs you can be on the look out for. In many cases, children who lose a parent will experience some going backward or stalling, in their developmental progress. While no two children grieve alike, there are some similarities for children who are in the same age group.

The ideas that follow are not meant to cover every grief reaction. Most children will go through a period of shock or disbelief and, as the reality that their parent is gone sinks in, they will feel a wide variety of feelings including sadness, anger, guilt, fear, and even relief. However, each child experiences and expresses their feelings about the death or loss of a parent differently.

For many children the loss of their parent will mean a drop in school performance. Caregivers, families, and the child can choose whether or not to talk to a child's teachers about the loss. If a family decides to speak with a teacher about the loss, they do not need to share the specifics about how the parent died. Before speaking with school personnel, the family may want to agree on a way to answer some questions about how the parent died. In many cases, a teacher who knows that one of their students has suffered a loss of this kind will make themselves more available to the child or at least keep a special eye on them.

Key Points about How Death Affects Children

1. It is age dependent
   —The very young, they need to understand that the body is not alive anymore and this is forever
   —Children seven to nine, the head knows, but it is hard to deal with the feelings and they begin to ask spiritual questions
   —Teens are hormone-driven and need to incorporate loss with all of their other feelings
2. Mourning comes and goes
3. They feel alone because our culture doesn't like to think or talk about death

Grieving Children Ask

1. Was it my fault?
2. Can I catch it?
3. Who will take care of me?

Children Two to Six Years Old

Common Reactions to Grief

- Increased reluctance to lose sight of the grandparent. They are more unsure and nervous about the world.
- Fears of the dark and "monsters." Often these children have trouble going to sleep and even become nervous when they see an adult sleeping.
- Loss of developmental achievements, such as toilet training.
- Difficulty with peers and a tendency to isolate themselves at school or in other group situations.
- More tantrums and refusals to do things that they used to accept without difficulty, like going to bed, eating, or putting on a coat.
- Difficulty concentrating in day care or school and during other activities.
- Feelings of guilt for the death of the parent. (Toddlers believe that their angry feelings for the deceased can have something to do with their death.)
- Blaming the surviving parent for the loss of the other.

When Grief Becomes Complicated

- Grief is persistent and pervasive for more than three months.
- The children isolate themselves from their peers and constantly cling to the grandparent.
- More than a year after the death, they are unable to concentrate on activities or school.

Try to:

- Allow the child to attend the funeral, visit the cemetery, and experience all the family rituals for grieving.
- Be simple, brief, and tell the truth when speaking about death.
- Say as many times as necessary that the death is not their fault, and reassure them of their health and yours.
- Help the child maintain an appropriate connection to their deceased parent by storytelling, drawing, or playing in ways that help them to express their grief. Do not be concerned if the child talks to his parent or says that the parent has spoken to him.
- Make sure the child has some items from the deceased parent that can be kept in a safe place.

Expect a return of grieving behaviors at special times such as birthdays, holidays, and the anniversary of the death.

Try to Avoid:

- Placing emotional expectations on the child, such as saying, "Why aren't you sadder?" or, "Stop crying, it's time to be a big boy now."
- Do not tell the child that the parent is asleep or that they are in a better place now.
- Expecting the child to be his or her "old self" too soon. Grieving takes time and there will be good and bad days for a while.

Seven- to Twelve-Year-Olds

Since many of these children understand that death is final, they may be unwilling to "believe" what has happened. Initially, they will probably be in shock, but with time they will begin to feel sad about their loss.

Some children will not do as well in school after their parent has died. However, this is usually temporary, and most children are able to return to their usual performance after approximately six months. This adjustment may take longer when the children have to move and change schools.

Common Reactions to Grief

- Headaches and stomachaches.
- Problems with sleeping, nightmares, and fear of the dark.
- Reluctance to play with friends and isolation at school and in the neighborhood.
- Temporary depression and hopelessness about their lives.

Signs That Grief is Complicated

- Makes no effort to spend time with friends (lasts more than six months).
- Poor school performance (lasts more than a year).
- Significant changes in appetite (lasts more than four months).
- Persistent sleep problems.
- Persistent headaches or stomachaches.
- Prolonged depression.
- Refusal to talk about the deceased parent.

Try to:

- Allow time for the reality of the death to "sink in" and make sure the child is invited to attend the funeral and participate in family grieving rituals.
- Respect the erratic grief of children; if they are upset one minute and playing the next, keep in mind that they are not being disrespectful, but are grieving in their own way.
- Make sure the child has mementos from the deceased parent.
- Reassure them that they did not do anything to cause their parent to leave.
- Allow the child to tell his/her best friend/friends/teachers, if they desire.

- Encourage normal life activities.
- Spend time with the child, telling stories and talking about the deceased parent.
- Encourage children to express themselves through drawing, stories, poems, and activities.

Try to Avoid:

- Pushing for feelings or expecting that their grieving will be short.
- Getting angry when the child seems to ignore the loss. Children's feelings come and go more rapidly than adults. They need time to play, even during the grieving process.
- Expecting them to return to their usual school performance level for about six months.

Thirteen- to Eighteen-Year-Olds

While one might think that the loss of a parent becomes easier as young people grow older, this is not necessarily true. There are many adolescents for whom the loss of a parent is very difficult, even when they did not have a very close relationship with that parent.

Teenagers often have difficulty talking about their feelings, or they are comfortable expressing only their anger and not their sadness and fear. This can be very frustrating for adults. It takes patience and caring for new caregivers to "hang in there" when a teenager is behaving badly and seems ungrateful. Teens were often trying to experiment with independence just when the parent left them. This makes independence even more confusing.

Common Reactions to Grief

- Anger, often directed at those who care about them the most.
- Decline in school performance and difficulty concentrating.
- Withdrawal from friends and regular activities.
- Brief periods of change in appetite and sleep.
- Headaches and stomachaches.
- Depression which is expressed through hopelessness.
- Feeling abandoned by the deceased parent.

Signs That Grief Is Complicated

- The teenager spends too much time avoiding their responsibilities: skipping school, not doing chores, etc.
- They use drugs/alcohol to "medicate" themselves against their grief.
- The adolescent never expresses any feelings concerning the deceased.
- Intense mood swings which last more than four months.
- School performance declines for longer than a year.
- Depression associated with the death lasts longer than three months.
- Frequent fights.

Try to:

- Talk as much as possible with the adolescent about the deceased, but do it during activities. This is much easier for adolescents to tolerate than face-to-face conversations.
- Give them permission, even encourage them, to talk to their peers about their loss.
- Include the adolescent in the planning and carrying-out of family rituals.
- Encourage them to express themselves by drawing, writing stories and poems.
- Encourage teenagers to stay in school and remind them that their ability to work and concentrate will return.

Try to Avoid:

- Pushing for feelings.
- Giving up when they test you. Do not give up on curfews or chores.
- Taking the angry or hurtful things they say too personally.

Even after the intense feelings of grief begin to subside, children will continue to want to hear stories about their parents. They need to hear the ways in which they are like their mothers and fathers, as well as the ways in which they are uniquely themselves. As the new caregiver, you have the opportunity to talk to them about the history that you know about their families. The more positive qualities and funny events you remember, the better. This helps children, and especially adolescents, begin to understand how they are like and not like their parents.

Helping Children Talk about Death

Death is a sensitive topic. Many adults feel uncomfortable explaining death honestly and openly to the children because of a desire to protect them from this or other painful issues that might arise.

Talking about death is a difficult thing to do, especially with young children. How do you feel about talking with the children? What is your own understanding of death? Have your religious or cultural beliefs helped you to talk to the children? Do you have an explanation of death that you feel comfortable using when you talk to the children? How did you tell them what happened to their parent? What have your discussions been like since the parent died?

It is certainly the grandparents' choice about how they want to explain the parent's death, but here are some general guidelines.

Because many of the children have seen their parent become sick and finally die, they may be afraid of illness in general, even the common cold. Reassure them of their safety by explaining the difference between an illness that is curable like the everyday cold, and illnesses which have no cure, but are rare and hard to get.

The death of a parent may cause children to feel unsure about the adults that are caring for them. Children need to be reassured that where they are living now is where they will remain.

If the grandparent is ill, it is important that he/she does not offer the children false hope about being able to take care of them forever. He/she might comfort the children by speaking in the here and now. *Reassure* the children by telling them that you are here to take care of them today and you will make sure that there will always be someone to take care of them in the future.

Making a Memory Box

If you have any souvenirs or pictures of the children with the parent, show them to the children—this might be a nice way to start conversations about what they remember. Consider starting a memory box (Brine & Lindsay-Smith, 1992), where each child holds things special to them. The child can choose what kind of box they want to use (shoe box, gift box, plastic box, lunch box, etc.). Begin by putting photos in it.

If you don't have any mementos of the past, this is a good time to start a memory box. You can keep school awards or report cards or new photos or greeting cards in it. The child will feel important because they have a place for special things. It can help them feel more special about themselves. It gives them a place to go to remember. You can also create a box or suitcase for yourself.

Activities

1) Role-play talking to a young child about loss and death.
2) Role-play talking to a teenager about loss and death.
3) Role-play what you would say to your grandchild if you became ill.

Session 10

Navigating the Service System

OUTLINE

A) Review of last session
B) Session objectives
C) Temporary Assistance to Needy Families (TANF)
D) Medicaid
E) Food Stamps
F) Supplemental Security Income (SSI)
G) Earned Income Tax Credit (EITC)
H) Getting through the system
I) Activities

Session 10

Navigating the Service System

Knowing how to get the services that you need for both yourself and your grandchild is a critical factor in becoming empowered. This really involves being able to navigate through an often very complex system. This navigation can be incredibly frustrating and tiring for everyone. This session offers tips and methods for learning how to effectively deal with agencies so that you can obtain the help that you need. Because program requirements change and often vary among the states, it is strongly suggested that a local agency person participate in this session.

Objectives

At the end of this session, participants will be able to:

1) Identify the services that can be important to grandparents raising grandchildren.
2) Describe ways of contacting these services.
3) Discuss why it is important to document agency contacts.
4) Explain the importance of "persistence" and "assertiveness."

There are many services that may assist you in caring for your grandchildren. These include Temporary Assistance to Needy Families (TANF), which has replaced Aid for Dependent Children (AFDC); Medicaid; Food Stamps; Supplementary Security Income (SSI); and Earned Income Tax Credit (EITC). The local Department of Social Services is the first place to contact for financial assistance. Payments are made on the basis of the child's income. The local office will tell you how to apply for benefits and food stamps and should also inform you about state and local programs that may assist you and your grandchild.

Temporary Assistance to Needy Families (TANF)

TANF provides cash assistance to grandparents caring for grandchildren on the basis of either your whole household income or your grandchild's income. Grandparents can apply as "caretaker relatives."

Grandparent-headed household (all family members receiving assistance:

- Must establish relationship to the grandchild, living arrangements, income, assets.
- Must meet asset requirements for your state.

Qualifying on behalf of grandchild:

- Grandchild must be under the age of eighteen.
- Must show that grandchild is without parental support due to death, absence, unemployment, or illness.
- Grandchild's income and assets must meet eligibility criteria.
- Grandparent must be "caretaker relative" which means that you must have proof that your grandchild is living in your home under your care.

Potential Problems

There may be problems proving that you are the "caretaker relative." You do not need to show legal custody of your grandchild. You only need to show that you are responsible for care, and prove that the child's parent is not providing care.

Medicaid

Medicaid is a national program funded by the federal government and state governments that provides medical assistance to persons with low incomes meeting eligibility criteria. Grandchildren may be eligible as either "categorically needy" or "medically needy."

Categorically Needy

- Grandchildren who receive TANF or SSI.
- Grandchildren who are eligible for TANF.
- Disabled grandchildren who do not qualify for SSI due to income may still be eligible for Medicaid.

Medically Needy

- Incomes are above the categorically needy level but are not sufficient to afford medical care.
- In order to receive Medicaid, grandparents may be asked to establish the child's paternity and to help obtain medical support from other insurance companies that may be involved in services for the child. You need to prove that you are the caretaker of the child but *do not* need to have legal custody. You will also have to show health insurance information although you do not need to have insurance information on the parent.

Potential Problems

If you receive TANF or SSI, you are automatically entitled to Medicaid. Workers may be reluctant or not know how to deal with the additional regulations involved in applications from those not receiving these benefits.

Food Stamps

Food stamps are available to low income people and families meeting state income and asset requirements.

They are issued monthly and the value is based on the number of persons in the household and household income.

To receive food stamps, the entire household must meet the eligibility requirements; this means grandparents, grandchildren, and anyone else living in the home.

The income on which food stamps are based includes many deductions which may make it easier for grandparents to be accepted into the program.

You do not need legal custody of your grandchild to receive food stamps.

Potential Problems

Because food stamps apply to the whole household, close attention needs to be paid to who in the home is actually part of the unit and who is not part of the grandparent-grandchild household. This can be complicated and workers will ask for documents related to this eligibility. If original documents are not available, you have to right to offer substitute documents.

Supplemental Security Income (SSI)

SSI is a national program offered through Social Security to low-income elderly, blind, or disabled persons.

Grandchildren can meet the requirements if they have a physical or mental disability which prevents them from doing things that other children their age do, are under eighteen years old, and fall below the income limits.

You may also qualify as a grandparent if you meet the income requirements.

Your income and assets are not included in determining your grandchild's eligibility for SSI, but your benefit may be reduced by one-third because the child is living in your home. However, if your grandchild is paying a "fair share" of the household expenses, the benefit may be increased.

If the benefit amount is less than the full federal benefit, you should insist on the "fair share" calculation. You have sixty days to challenge the benefit you are given.

Your grandchild *cannot* receive both TANF and SSI so you must assess which is best for your situation.

Applications are made at the local Social Security office. If you receive a letter that you or your grandchild are not eligible, you have the right to know why. You then have sixty days to appeal. SSA has a toll-free hotline to find out about the appeal process: 1-800-772-1213.

Potential Problems

1) Demonstrating that you are responsible for your grandchild; you do not have to have legal custody.
2) Proving that the grandchild has a disability which meets the standard.
3) Receiving the maximum benefit to which your grandchild is entitled.

Earned Income Tax Credit (EITC)

This is a benefit for low-income and moderate-income working persons who are raising children. It provides working grandparents with additional income through a cash payment. The amount is based on a percentage of the grandparent's earnings.You do not have to have legal custody of your grandchild.

Grandparents must file an income tax return to receive this benefit.

Your earned income during the year must have fallen below the established limits, but this does not include Social Security benefits, TANF payments, pensions, or other benefits.

Grandchild must be under the age of nineteen, under the age of twenty-four and a full-time student, or disabled.

A proportion of the total benefit, 60%, can be received weekly, biweekly, or monthly, or the total can be received as a refund at the end of the year.

To receive the regular payments, an IRS form W-5 must be filed with the employer so that the amount is figured in with the paycheck.

You and your grandchild must have lived in the same home for more than six months.

It is important to note that the EITC is not counted as income when applying for other public benefits.

Getting Through the System

Applying for public benefits can be frustrating and time-consuming. You should expect to make at least two visits. Bring as much information with you as you can, including:

1) The grandchild's birth certificate
2) The parent's birth certificate to prove your relationship to the child
3) Social Security numbers for everyone in the family
4) Proof of income for everyone in the family (pay stubs, SS payments, child support stubs)
5) Proof of assets for everyone in family (bank statements, house deed, car title)
6) Document which shows you are the "caretaker relative" of your grandchild

Be Organized

On the Telephone:

- Before you go, get as much information as possible about the program.
- Make as many telephone calls as necessary, don't give up.
- Keep records of your telephone calls and be sure to get names and titles of those you speak with.
- Take notes on the telephone. You may repeat these notes to the person to make sure you are correct.

At the Agency:

- Be on time for your appointment. Bring someone with you if it will make you feel more comfortable.
- Have all of your documents in a folder so that they are readily available.
- Write down questions and concerns before your meeting to make sure they are addressed.
- Take notes if you need to during the meeting.
- At the end of a meeting or conversation, review your notes and confirm with the person what the next step will be and who will make it.

After the Meeting:

- If you believe you are not getting what you need, ask to speak to the supervisor. If this is not helpful, insist on speaking with the manager, agency director, etc.
- Go through the proper channels and do not be afraid of moving up the ladder. Be assertive but not aggressive.
- Keep documents to show the course that you have taken.
- It may be most effective to call in the morning between 7 and 9 or in the late afternoon (after 5) as supervisors often answer the phones at these times.
- Keep trying and don't be afraid to call back if you are denied assistance. Talk to people who have been through the system and get tips from them. Ask questions and don't give up!

Be Assertive

- Learn not to take "no" for an answer.
- Do not lose your temper even though you are losing your patience.
- Stay calm and persistent—this may mean repeating your request several times or demanding to speak to another staff person.
- Knowing your rights is important as a basis for your demand.
- Be clear about what you seek and why you believe you are entitled to it.
- Remember you may know more than the agency person.

Obtaining Needed Documents

Birth certificates—Contact the Bureau of Vital Statistics in the state and county of your grandchild's birth. You may need to have a court order to gain permission to get the certificate.

Medical records—Parents should be contacted for the records. Their pediatrician's office or clinic may also help. If your grandchild has been enrolled in school, the school may give you a copy.

You may also:

- Make a list of all medical conditions or illnesses you remember your grandchild having.
- List the medical history of the child's parents, including medical conditions of the mother during pregnancy.

Activities

---

1) Describe public benefit programs available to grandparents and grandchildren.
2) Role-play a telephone call to an agency asking for assistance.
3) Role-play actions to take when a person is not cooperative or denies you benefits to which you believe you are eligible.

Session 11

Legal and Entitlement Issues

OUTLINE

A) Review of last session
B) Session objectives
C) Reasons to plan
D) Using a lawyer
E) Legal options for permanency planning
F) Wills
G) Activities
H) Legal resources

Session 11

Legal and Entitlement Issues

Keeping track of you and your grandchild's legal and entitlement issues may feel like a full-time job. The legal system is very complicated and having a lawyer to help you understand and sort through your options can be helpful. Legal help is available through local legal aid programs as well as through private attorneys. Area Agencies on Aging or Departments on Aging should be able to offer assistance in locating legal advice.

Objectives

At the end of this session, participants will be able to:

1) Assess whether you have the best legal plan for you and your grandchild.
2) Describe the different types of living arrangements.
3) Discuss the role of wills in planning for the future.
4) Know where to get free legal assistance.

It is helpful to have a local attorney present during this session since many areas require interpretation and laws differ considerably among the states.

Arrangements for the Care of Grandchildren

Informal Arrangements

These arrangements are without any legal status and, consequently, the grandparent's relationship with the grandchild is neither secure nor binding. These arrangements suggest that the care is only temporary, rather than final, and that the situation is likely to change. However, the informality also means:

1) The grandparents have no legal status in any dispute with the parents or any officials.
2) The grandparent may not have legal documents necessary for making decisions for schools or medical care.
3) An inability to obtain benefits and types of assistance for raising the grandchild.
4) Problems in obtaining health insurance for the grandchild.

Legal Arrangements

Legal relationships are the only ways to assure that a grandparent's decision-making authority over the grandchild is secure. Going through the legal process can be complex and difficult and may involve court proceedings. In going through any legal proceedings, it is always best to have a qualified lawyer who is familiar with your type of situation. There are several types of legal arrangements that secure the relationship between grandparents and grandchildren.

1) Adoption

This process affords the grandparent the same legal rights and duties to the grandchild as that of the parent. It usually involves the complete termination of the parents' rights to the child. It involves going to court and having the court investigate the grandparents to determine if they are fit to adopt. Adoption assures the children of a permanent home.

a) The court must show that adoption is in the best interest of the child.
b) After the application is filed, the court considers the investigative report and decides whether to approve the adoption.
c) If approved, the parents' rights are terminated and grandparents assume all rights and responsibilities, including financial support.
d) If eligible, grandparents may receive public benefits.
e) Adoptive grandparents are not eligible for foster care payments, but some children who have been in foster care are eligible for subsidies.
f) In many states, foster parents have priority in adopting the child.

2) *Guardianship*

Guardianship is a formal legal relationship established by a court which gives the grandparent the authority to make decisions for the child due to the parent's absence or incapacity. Types of guardianships include legal guardianship, standby guardianship, joint guardianship, and testamentary guardianship. These are not available in every state and therefore it is important to learn what is possible in your area.

Legal Guardianship

- Appointed by a judge when it is found to be in best interest of child.
- Parental rights are suspended, not terminated.
- Parents responsible for support of the children.
- Parents cannot remove children from home without guardian's permission.
- With legal guardianship, grandparents are able to:

  1) Make decisions regarding care of grandchildren including school enrollment and medical care.
  2) Apply for public benefits.
  3) Pursue child support payments from parents.

Standby Guardianship

Authorizes parents to designate the grandparent to become the legal guardian when they are not able to care for the children. The court is not required to approve this guardian, so it is best to have the person appointed as standby before the parent's death or incapacity. Parents can decide when the guardianship becomes effective.

Testamentary Guardianship

Parents name a guardian in their will and are recommending that this person become the children's guardian when they die. There is no guarantee that the court will appoint that person, as it must decide that the appointment will be in the child's best interest. It is less useful than a standby guardianship, but if the standby is not available in the state, this is one way of planning for the children's future care.

Powers of Attorney

These documents authorize the grandparent to be able to make decisions on behalf of the children when the parents are absent or unable to do so. In some states, these rights are limited to a specific period of time. Powers of Attorney permit the grandparents to make school or medical decisions without being the guardian. Parental rights are not terminated and they still have legal custody of the children.

Foster Care

In some cases, the child welfare agency has legal custody of the child either because the parent has voluntarily placed the child with the agency or because the agency has removed the child from the home.

Grandparents may become foster parents to the grandchild and thus eligible for a foster care subsidy.

1) Foster care is expected to be temporary, but if the parent does not resume care in a specified time, their rights may be terminated. As foster parents, grandparents are eligible for a foster care subsidy to help support the child. If grandparents become legal guardians or adopt the child, these subsidies stop.

2) The child welfare agency has custody and the grandparent foster parents report to the agency. The grandparents do not have the right to make medical decisions for the child and the agency can remove the child from the home if it is felt to be unsuitable.

3) If the court determines the parents are able to care for the child, the child will be returned to the parents. If not, the parents' rights may be terminated and the child made eligible for adoption.

4) You cannot change from being a guardian to a foster parent but you can transfer from foster parent to guardian.

5) As a foster parent, you must be certified or licensed by the child welfare agency.

Will

A will (also financial instrument) is a document stating your wishes about what you want to happen after your death.

1) It is best to have an attorney to assist in making the will.
2) A will says who you want to assume guardianship of your grand-children. A court would take this as one factor in deciding guardianship.
3) It states where your property and possessions should go.
4) It pays your debts.
5) Your wishes about a funeral and burial are stated in the will.
6) Someone is appointed to carry out your wishes stated in the will (executor).
7) A will appoints a trustee to administer any trusts.

Activities
---

1) Describe the different types of guardianship.
2) Role-play discussing foster care with a grandparent.
3) Discuss the purposes that a will fulfills.

Legal Resources—National Organizations

The following organizations maintain information on current laws and legal assistance available to grandparents, including links to local resources.

American Bar Association
Center on Children and the Law
or
Commission on Legal Problems of the Elderly
740 15th Street NW
Washington, DC 20005
Tel. (202) 662-1000

Brookdale Center on Aging
Grandparent Caregiver Law Center
425 East 25th Street, 9th Floor
New York, NY 10010
Tel. (212) 481-4433

American Bar Association
750 N. Lake Shore Drive
Chicago, IL 60611
Tel. (312) 988-5000

Session 12

Developing Advocacy Skills

OUTLINE

A) Review of last session
B) Session objectives
C) Outreach activities
D) Making contacts
E) Key officials
F) Lobbying and political action
G) Writing letters
H) Activities

Session 12

Developing Advocacy Skills

A dvocacy involves the activities you undertake to make your needs as grandparents known. Learning the necessary skills for being effective advocates will help to assure that you get your message clearly through to others, so that appropriate policies and services to meet your needs can be developed. Effective advocacy can also involve expanding your own group. As participation grows, the group becomes more noticeable to community leaders and policy makers and thus can have can have more impact in forcing change. It is important to remember that advocacy involves the use of power, and power depends on factors such as knowledge of issues and problems, participants, respect, and solidarity.

Objectives

At the end of this session, participants will be able to:

1) Discuss the types of outreach they can do as grandparents.
2) Explain ways of contacting persons who can provide needed information or assistance.
3) Demonstrate their skills in telephoning and writing letters to community leaders in order to get their needs met.
4) Discuss ways of making their needs known.

Outreach Activities

Outreach refers to all of the activities you might do to reach others in the community for a specific purpose. This may include recruiting new members to the support group or educating community leaders and others about your activities or needs.

The first step in outreach is to decide whom it is you want to contact and what it is you want to contact them about. For example, if you want to bring more members into the group, you might want to hand out brochures that describe the group to persons who look like they may be grandparents. If you want to educate community leaders and others about your activities or need, you might want to hold a community event like an open house or workshop at your church.

Community Event

The community event is an important way to publicize your group and your activities. It can be very helpful in attracting new participants as well as a way for distributing information to other grandparents. The event can also be important in helping you to make contacts and act as a basis for making community change. The event establishes your group in the community by giving it real visibility.

Steps to Take

1) Decide first on the theme of the event. It could simply be, "Making Grandparents Aware of Services and Rights."
2) After the theme is decided, invite speakers to present at the workshop. Speakers could include a lawyer, a teacher, someone from the local government, a social worker, and, definitely, a grandparent. They should be knowledgeable about the needs of grandparents and their grandchildren and be able to present information in a lively and engaging way.
3) Publicize the event in local newspapers, churches, schools, and community calendars.

4) Locate community persons who will help to promote the event. Be sure to invite local officials and council members to the event. These persons like being seen in the community and it promotes the organization.

Participation in Community Programs

Another way to publicize your activities and to reach other grandparents is to participate in community programs or events that are being held. Community centers, neighborhoods, and churches often have fairs in which groups set up their own booths. Staffing the booth with grandparents and giving out brochures on your group, as well as answering questions, are immediate ways of reaching others.

Reaching Out

One of the easiest ways to do outreach is through direct contact, reaching out, to other persons. Talking directly to others who appear to be grandparents, and giving them information or brochures are very direct ways of making contact. As an example, at the doctor's office you might see a person who appears to be a grandparent with a child, and start telling them a little bit about your situation and the group you belong to. Each of you will have your own way of starting a conversation, but, *remember*, the goal of meeting is to help the person and to get him or her interested in your group.

Making Contacts

Joining Coalitions

Contacts are often made with other agencies or groups. Sometimes it is helpful to join with other programs in seeking particular goals. This type of coalition can be very effective in getting your own message heard as well as in effecting change since there is more power in the numbers represented by the coalition. However, it is important to be sure that you and the other members of the coalition have similar values and aims and that you can respect one another as you work together.

- Decide which agencies or programs share similar interests with your own.
- Are there other groups of grandparents in the community?
- What about other groups such as women's groups connected with a church or social agencies? Would they be interested in meeting with your group monthly to discuss issues and ways of getting changes in policies and services?
- Other groups that might be interested in joining include teachers, counselors, police, clergy, youth groups, city council members and other persons who are involved with children.
- Groups that work with older persons and families such as senior centers and services, counseling agencies, and educational programs may also be interested in joining with you.

Individuals in Key Positions

These are the persons who have the power and authority to make change happen and who can be instrumental in helping you to achieve your goals.

First, decide who these persons are. Often, they are persons in the neighborhood who don't have an official title but who are able to get things done! They are the persons people turn to for help.

Depending on the specific issue, these key persons could be in the schools, health care programs, social service agencies, or local councils. As an example, if you are advocating for more school counseling for children, the key persons may be the school principals and the school board, who control funds. If you want a change in custody procedures, you might approach a council member.

When Approaching the Key Official, It Is Helpful to:

1) Know your facts—as an example, you might need to describe the problems that grandchildren are experiencing and the stress it is placing on grandparents.

2) Be specific in what you want—as examples, school counseling that is sensitive to the special problems of grandchildren, after-school programs, or custody proceedings that always include the grandparents.

3) Write down all of your questions and concerns before the meeting to make sure that you don't forget anything. You can refer to the list during the meeting if necessary.

4) Have your materials organized (papers, forms, brochures, etc.) so that you can easily refer to them or hand them out.

5) Listen carefully, take notes, and ask questions.

6) Before the meeting ends, try to reach a clear decision about, or understanding of what will happen next.

Telephone Contacts

When telephoning, give your name and the name of the grandparents' group or program that you represent. Example: "Hello, my name is Mary Walker and I am with the Grandparents Movement. I would like to speak with Mr. Pierce."

Lobbying and Political Actions

1) Get to know your local council members and legislators. Invite these persons to a meeting to share with them information and your concerns. Often, the best time is for coffee in the morning, before they get too busy with other meetings.

2) It is a good idea to also contact them when they do something you like—"Fan Mail." This will be remembered and can be important when you feel you need them for something else.

3) Prepare for the meeting, learn as much as possible about the council members and their views. Be clear about what it is that you want to discuss and share with them what it is you would like changed.

4) Attend public meetings and ask questions about officials' positions on issues which concern grandparents. *Don't be shy about*

raising your hand! Give your name and the name of the group that you represent. The more grandparents do this, the more officials will take notice of them and understand that the issue is important in the community.

a) Be sure to speak clearly and slowly.

b) Get right to the point, you usually have no more than two or three minutes.

c) State your concern and ask what the officials' views or plans in dealing with it are.

d) If the person is not familiar with the problem, invite him or her to a meeting so they can learn more about it.

Writing Letters

Letter writing can be important in making your needs known. The first decision must be who to write to. If the concern affects many grandparents, it can be particularly powerful to have everyone write similar letters to the same person. This helps to demonstrate that the problem is widespread. The letter should state the reason that you are writing, what the concern or issue is, and what you would like done.

Sample Letter

If possible, this should be on letterhead stationery of the group or organization. Typing is helpful, but legibility is most important.

Councilman Robert Robinson
110 West 125th Street
New York, NY 11111

Dear Councilman Robinson,

As a grandparent raising two grandchildren in your district, I have a very deep and personal interest in improving services for these children. There are more than 5,000 children living with their grandparents in this area and many of them are in need of . . . As a member of the "XYZ" Grandparent group, I have seen first hand the needs of these grandchildren.

Under the current law, these children are not entitled to . . . However, this causes many problems for grandparents who are trying very hard to make ends meet and to keep these children out of the formal child welfare system. I am asking your help in developing policies which will make it easier for grandparents to care of their grandchildren. We need programs such as . . .

Our grandchildren are very important to us and we want to make sure that everything possible is done to help them to adjust to their situations. We would very much like you to come to one of our meetings so that we can talk with you further about our plans.

Thank you very much. I look forward to hearing from you.

Sincerely,

Mary Carter

Mary Carter
222 West 111th Street
New York, NY 11111
(212) 555-1111

Activities

---

1) Role-play the way in which you might approach a grandparent in the community to inform her or him about your program.
2) Role-play a telephone call to a local official that you are making on behalf of your program in order to get support.
3) Role-play speaking out at a public meeting on services for grandparents.

Session 13

Getting Your Message Across

OUTLINE

A) Review of last session
B) Session objectives
C) Preparing for a presentation
D) Starting a presentation
E) Main points of the presentation
F) The closing
G) Activities

Session 13

Getting Your Message Across

You may be asked to give presentations on your group, on your experiences as a grandparent, on your activities, or on many different issues. The purpose of this session is to help you to both enjoy these presentations and to make them as effective as possible in getting your message across. This session should include several opportunities to try out the different suggestions.

Objectives

At the end of this session, participants will be able to:

1) Describe how to prepare for a presentation.
2) Know how to get their message across.
3) Understand the importance of body language, eye contact, and voice.
4) How to relax before a speech.

Preparing for a Presentation

The first step in preparing for a presentation is to learn about your audience; who are you talking to? Your presentation is going to be different depending on whether you are talking to children, grandparents, or community officials. There will be different reasons for people coming to your presentation—out of interest, because they were told to come, because they know you and want to help. Having an idea of why they are there will help you in preparing the talk. *How much does the audience know?* Don't waste people's time by telling them things they already know. But, if they don't know, you must teach them or help them to understand that they need to know more about grandparents and grandchildren.

Rehearse

Go over what you are going to say so that you know the material. Say the whole speech out loud at least once. Don't try to memorize, just rehearse how you are going to talk so that you are comfortable.

Have Notes

Write down your main points so you are sure to get them across. You don't have to have the whole speech written out. Cards are better than paper.

Dressing for the Presentation

Dress nicely. A bright scarf can bring attention to your face. Be comfortable in your clothes and wear what makes you feel good. Don't wear noisy chains or bracelets.

Eye Contact

Eye contact is important and powerful. Look at one person in the audience, then turn to someone else on the other side of the room. This makes people feel that they have contact with you.

Voice

- Be sure you are loud enough to be heard.
- Don't' talk too fast or too slow.
- Pause in your talk to give people time to think about what you are saying.

Relaxing Before the Presentation

- Shut your eyes, let your head droop forward. Inhale slowly, turn your head to the right, exhale and let it droop forward again. Inhale and do the same thing turning to the left.
- Inhale and let your head rotate all around and then reverse (making circles with your head).
- Imagine yourself doing it well, people hearing you and agreeing, and imagine yourself being self-assured!!
- Take a few deep breaths before you begin and keep breathing.
- Believe in the importance of what you are saying and its purpose.

Starting a Presentation

Get the group's attention: You might want to start with a very short story that connects you with the group. "Most of us have had grandparents and most of us will be grandparents, but let me tell you there is a lot to know and be prepared for . . . it isn't all hugs and kisses . . . its also tears and anger . . . "

Establish yourself as a person who knows: You may need to briefly describe your role as a grandparent, your background . . . "As a grandmother raising three grandchildren, ages two, four, and five for the last three years, I want to share with you some of the important issues to be faced . . . "

Depending on you audience, you might want to give some statistics such as the number of grandparents raising grandchildren in the community, the reasons for this, and the problems they face. Be brief with your introduction; once people know who you are and that you know the facts, it's time to get on with the message. Taking too much time in the introduction will lose the audience.

The Body of the Talk

People are with you now so give them your message:

> "I'd like to tell you about the group I belong to and what it can do for you . . . "
>
> "I'm here to ask for your help and support in getting more services for grandparents . . . "
>
> "It is time for the members of this community to stand up to the . . . and demand more . . . "

Main Points of Presentation

People never remember more than five key points, so keep it simple. Often, you start with your most important point:
Example: In a presentation to community leaders for more services:

> Grandmothers are raising more and more grandchildren because of the problems that are attacking our community and our children. Drugs, AIDS, and crime are having serious effects on our neighborhood and we are now becoming responsible for raising our grandchildren. We are accepting this responsibility because these are our babies and our first concern is keeping them out of the child welfare system. But, raising them means that we are . . . (describe the effects, problems, etc.).

Next, state what you need or propose:

> To take care of these grandchildren we need more services and more help such as . . .

State how getting what you propose will improve the situation:

> By getting these services and programs, these grandchildren will have a better chance of succeeding in school and in the community. As grandparents, we

will be able to feel secure that they are going to grow up to be responsible and caring adults.

Tell people what you want them to do:
(You've told them what is needed and why so now you have to tell them exactly what you want.)

I'm asking that you give more funds for . . . I'm asking you to come to our group and see what we're all about . . .

The Closing

- End on time—don't go on too long; know how long you have to speak and stick to it. People get tired and restless listening and you don't want to lose them at the end.
- Tell people you are ending: *"In conclusion,"* or *"I want to end by saying . . . "*
- Summarize and emphasize your main ideas:

In conclusion, grandparents are raising their grandchildren and are happy to do it—but, we need services and help so that we can do it well and make sure that our grandchildren grow to be successful and responsible adults . . .

- Don't add any new points here, but you might want to tell people where they can get more information about your group.
- End with a bang—make sure the ending is strong. It is the last thing the group hears and you want them to remember. You could ask for action:

Now is the time to talk to the school board. At tomorrow night's meeting, speak out about the need for after-school programs for our grandchildren.

- You can also end with a question:

These are our children, can we afford not to help them?

- Send the people home thinking about what you have said, what needs to be done, and what they can do.

Activities

1) Role-play a five minute presentation to a group of grandmothers about the importance of joining a support group.
2) Role-play a five minute presentation to a group of community leaders about the need for more after-school programs.
3) Role-play different types of endings to a presentation.

Session 14

What Did We Learn?

The purpose of this training course was to provide material that can help to empower you both within your family and within the community. You should now be better able to deal with the issues involved in raising your grandchildren. You should also feel more comfortable in reaching out to other grandparents and to those responsible for policies and services that affect you. This session will review the topics that have been covered and explore which areas you feel require further discussion.

Objectives

1) To review the previous classes.
2) To identify the most helpful or useful points in each of the classes.
3) To identify the areas where more learning is needed.
4) To identify the areas that were least helpful.

Activities

1) Participants will discuss the topics they felt most helpful and explain why.

2) Participants will discuss the areas where more learning is needed.
3) Participants will discuss the areas that were least helpful and explain why.
4) Course evaluations will be completed.

References and Resources

American Association of Retired Persons. (1995). *Tips for grandparents: Finding help untangling the web of public programs.* Washington, DC: Author.

Berger, P., & Neuhaus, R. (1977). *To empower people: The role of mediating structures in public policy.* Washington, DC: American Enterprise Institute for Public Policy Research.

Brine, R., & Lindsay-Smith, C. (1992). *The memory store and memory book.* Essex, England: Barnardo.

City of New York, Department of Aging. Grandparent Resource Center. (1996). *For grandparents raising grandchildren: A series of workshops to help you cope.* New York: Author.

Cochran, M. (1987). Empowering families: An alternative to the deficit model. In K. Hurrelman, F. Kaufman, and Losel, (Eds.), *Social intervention: Potential and constraints* (pp. 105–119). Berlin: Walter de Bruyter.

The DC Kinship Care Coalition, Inc. (1996). *The Kinship Care Source Book.* Washington, DC: Author.

DiClemente, C., & Norcross, J. (1992). In search of how people change. *American Psychologist, 47,* 1102–1114.

Generations United. (1998). *Grandparents and Other Relatives Raising Children: An Intergenerational Action Agenda.* Washington, DC: Author.

Gutierrez, L. (1990). Working with women of color: An empowerment perspective. *Social Work, 35,* 149–154.

Gutierrez, L., & Ortega, R. (1991). Developing methods to empower Latinos: The importance of groups. *Social Work with Groups, 14,* 23–43.

Hasenfeld, Y. (1987). Power in social work practice. *Social Service Review, 61,* 467–483.

Illinois Department on Aging. (1999). *Starting points for grandparents raising grandchildren.* Springfield: Author.

Katz, R. (1984). Empowerment synergy: Expanding the community's healing resources. *Prevention in Human Services, 3,* 9–36.

Lee, J. (1994). *The empowerment approach to social work practice.* New York: Columbia University Press.

Lowy, L., & O'Connor, D. (1986). *Why Education in the Later Years.* Lexington: Lexington Books.

Prochaska, J. (1995). Common problems: Common solutions. *Clinical Psychology: Science and Practice, 2.*

Staples, L. (1990). Powerful ideas about empowerment. *Administration in Social Work, 14,* 29–42.

National Organizations

These national organizations focus on the needs of grandparent caregivers and their grandchildren. They can provide current information on policies and services.

American Association of Retired Persons
Grandparent Information Center
601 E Street NW
Washington, DC 20049
Tel. (202) 434-2296

American Bar Association
Center on Children and the Law
740 15th Street NW
Washington, DC 20005
Tel. (202) 662-1000

Brookdale Center on Aging
Grandparent Caregiver Law Center
425 East 25th Street, 9th Floor
New York, NY 10010
Tel. (212) 481-4433

The Brookdale Foundation Group
125 East 56th Street
New York, NY 10022
Tel. (212) 308-7355

Children's Defense Fund
25 E Street NW
Washington, DC 20001
Tel. (202) 628-8787

Child Welfare League of America
Cultural Competence and Kinship Care Services
440 First Street, Suite 310
Washington, DC 20001
Tel. (202) 638-2952

G.A.P. (Grandparents As Parents)
C/O Sylvie de Toledo
P.O. Box 964
Lakewood, CA 90714
Tel. (562) 924-3996

Generations United
440 First Street, 4th Floor
Washington, DC 20001
Tel. (202) 662-4283

Grandparents for Grandparents, Inc.
P.O. Box 42
Whitehouse Station, NJ 08889
Tel. (908) 534-4961

Grandparents' Rights Organization
100 West Long Lake Road, Suite 250
Bloomfield Hills, MI 48304
Tel. (248) 646-7191

National Coalition of Grandparents
Central Headquarters
137 Larkin Street
Madison, WI 53705
Tel. (608) 238-8751

National Committee to Preserve Social Security and Medicare
2000 K Street NW, Suite 800
Washington, DC 20006
Tel. (202) 966-1935

National Council on the Aging
409 Third Street SW, Suite 200
Washington, DC 20024
Tel. (202) 479-1200

ROCKING Inc. (Raising Our Children's Kids: An Intergenerational
Network of Grandparenting, Inc.)
P.O. Box 96
Niles, MT 49120
Tel. (616) 833-7200

Index

Acting out, 30
Action, in stages of change, 16
Active learning, 3
Adolescents:
  behavior problems in, 43
  disclosure of illness, 33
  drug discussions, 58
  grief reactions, 78–80
  HIV discussions, 52
  responses to painful news, 30
  sex discussions, 48
Adoption, 96–97
Advocacy:
  importance of, 5, 103
  skills development, *see* Advocacy
    skills
Advocacy skills, development of:
  contacts, 105–107
  letter-writing guidelines, 108–109
  lobbying and political actions,
    107–108
  outreach activities, 104–105
  role-playing exercises, 118
  session objectives, 102
Aggressive behavior, 41
Alcohol, discussions guidelines, 56
Alienation, 69
American Association of Retired Persons, 123
American Bar Association, contact information, 100, 123
Anger, nature of, 43–44

Area Agencies on Aging, 95
Arrangements for care of grandchildren:
  adoption, 96–97
  foster care, 98–99
  guardianship, legal, 97–98
  informal, 96
Attention-getters, in presentations, 115

Bad language, 41–42, 44
Bed-wetting, 30
Behavior changes, implications of, 30,
  40–41
Behavior problems, dealing with:
  in adolescents, 43
  anger, nature of, 43–44
  misbehavior, prevention strategies,
    39–40
  painful news, response to, 30
  punishment, discipline distinguished
    from, 40–41
  questions to ask, 38–39
  session objectives, 37
  spanking, 40
  in young children, 41–43
Birth certificates, obtaining, 92
Birth control, 50–51
Biting behavior, 41
Blame, in grieving process, 75
Brochures, as information resource, 3
Broken rules, response to, 21, 39–40,
  48, 57